Yoga of Nature

Yoga of Nature
Union with Fire, Earth, Air & Water

Thia Luby

*For my sister Pam &
family)
Try these yoga poses
for a new refreshing
life!
I love you all,
Thia Luby
July 13, 2004*

Clear Light Publishing
Santa Fe, New Mexico

DEDICATION & ACKNOWLEDGMENTS

This book is dedicated to all my relatives who watched me blossom away from the normal path of our family. To my brother Gordie who was my mentor and my first introduction to yoga. . . . I miss you. To my Aunt Tillie, Aunt Irma and my parents, Edwin and Amelia Lineberger, who devoted their lives to teaching and always aspired to become writers. To my daughter, Bianca, and her husband, Chris, who now have my two beautiful grandchildren, Gage and Jazmyn, to raise. To my sister, Pam, and her children, Jeff, Brian and Lisa, and to my brother Greg. This is a celebration to honor all your influences in my life, helping me to become the teacher and writer of the family. Thank you from the bottom of my heart. Life is beautiful.

I wish to thank all who helped to make this book possible, especially the El Gancho Fitness, Swim & Racquet Club and its owner, Bill Sisneros. I also wish to thank my students, who patiently posed for and graciously allowed all the pictures to be included. The adult students are Samantha Garcia, Astrid Kuipers, Heidi Lyons, Sage Paisner and Michael Warren. The children are Peter Bessone, Stephany Bonifer, Isabella Ariel Coppler, Charlotte Casey, Grant Duke and Dolna Smithback. Thank you all for your patience, devotion and understanding in helping me photograph the images this book.

©2004 Thia Luby
Clear Light Publishing, 823 Don Diego Avenue, Santa Fe, New Mexico 87505
www.clearlightbooks.com

First Edition
10 9 8 7 6 5 4 3 2 1

Library of Congress Cataloging-in-Publication Data

Luby, Thia, 1954–
    Yoga of nature: union with fire, earth, air & water / by Thia Luby.—
1st ed.
             p. cm.
    Includes bibliographical references.
    ISBN 1-57416-073-7 (pbk.)
    1. Yoga—Popular works. I. Title.
    RA781.7.L8163 2003
    613.7'046—dc21

                                                                    2002156511

Outdoor photograph on page 40 ©Daniel Valdes. Photographs of Thia Luby on pages 2, 3, 5 (lower photo), 8, 9, 11, 14 (right), 15, 18, 19, 23, 24, 26, 27, 28, 29, 30, 38, 39, 44, 45, 46, 49, 51, 53 (w. Astrid), 55, 57, 59, 61, 63, 65, 67, 69, 71, 82, 88, 89, 101 and 102 ©Daniel Valdes. Photograph of bonfire on page XII, Navajoland mesa on page 20 and Thia Luby on page 122 ©Marcia Keegan. Photograph of ocean on page 72 ©Carol O'Shea. All other photographs and illustration on page X ©Thia Luby.

Book interior design/typography/production: Carol O'Shea, Cover design: Marcia Keegan/Carol O'Shea, Front cover photograph of Thia Luby ©Daniel Valdes.

The author and publisher accept no responsibility or liability for injuries that may result from use of the information in this book. Readers are expected to follow recommended precautions and make allowances for differences in abilities and physical condition. As is the case for all exercise programs, persons should check with their medical practitioners before beginning work on yoga poses.

Printed in Korea.

Table of Contents

INTRODUCTION

BALANCING THE ELEMENTS OF OUR NATURE

The four elements that form the macrocosm of our existence on Earth—fire, earth, air and water—maintain a balance and harmony that allow life to continue. Similarly, the individual body/mind needs to maintain balance and harmony. Practicing yoga by drawing on all four elements helps bring us into balance and harmony with the life cycle.

Fire poses are used to produce heat and light in various areas of the body for inner strength and stability. Fire refers to the fire of digestion and elimination that re-creates the body every day and gives us vital energy. It also relates to light entering areas of the body that are heavy or blocked internally, such as the heart, throat and head. This light clears energy blocks.

Earth poses relate to the most solid parts of our body and the way we are affected by gravity.

Grounding energy is brought downward through different parts of the body when connecting to the earth—the feet, buttocks, hands or head.

Air poses relate to breathing and *prana*, the energy of breath, as well as to the constellations that give us a larger sense of the universe. The *pranayama* (breathing exercises) increase oxygen in the body to help clear the mind, stimulate the brain and strengthen the lungs and heart. The poses relating to the sun-sign constellations bring us closer to our own personal power and take the focus off ourselves, placing it instead on the bigger picture, uniting us with the universe.

Water poses reflect the fact that we are mostly water, which enables us to flow and be flexible. Water animals are models for some of these poses; through these poses we may learn the animals'

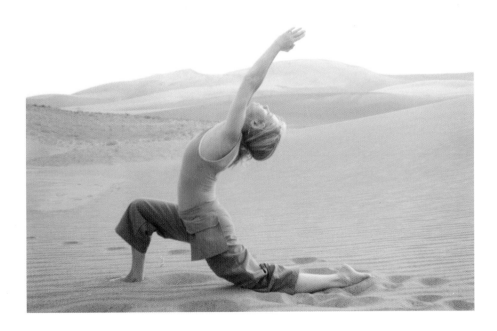

ability to float through life, free of burdens. Water poses also include waves for experiencing the ebb and flow of life and keeping the spine flexible. These balance out the nervous system.

To gain a clear understanding of how all the elements affect yoga practice, I urge you to read through the entire book before exploring the nature poses. At the back of the book you will find several chapters treating in detail subjects mentioned briefly in the rest of the text. For example, the chapter titled "The Science of Yoga" (p. 97) outlines the theory of yoga and *prana* (energy) and provides information on the eight limbs of *raja* yoga, which you can consciously practice to enrich every minute of your life. "The Chakra System" (p. 103) shows how the seven primary chakras relate to the poses and to the organs and glands that are stimulated during practice. In "Healing the Body/Mind — Yoga Therapy" (p. 107), you will find information on the connection between the physical and emotional bodies as well as recommended poses and breathing practices for dealing with common imbalances. Combining the guidance in these chapters with careful practice of the nature poses will enhance your life both physically and spiritually.

The book also provides lists of poses for strengthening and stretching different parts of the body, together with sample workouts graded according to difficulty. To create your own balanced workout for opening energy blocks throughout the body, first read through the book and practice enough poses from the different elements to help you clearly understand your own needs, strengths and weaknesses. Then pick one or more poses from each category.

Yoga practice is designed to help us tune into our bodies, unite body and mind and feed our *prana*, or life energy. In practicing yoga, we learn to relieve stress and become more sensitive to our needs, balancing out our strengths and weaknesses. We discover our true nature by delving deeply into how we feel and who we are.

Yoga helps us feel more alive. As you continue your practice, it is natural to lengthen your practice sessions, because the body/mind likes to feel good and craves a daily energy boost. Enjoy this unique blending of yoga with the elements of nature and see how your practice enhances your life. Regular practice of yoga is the best medicine for any aching body or soul.

"(Yoga is) wisdom in work or skillful living amongst activities, harmony and moderation. The yoga poses keep the body healthy and strong and in harmony with nature. He (the yogi) conquers the body and renders it a fit vehicle for the soul. This leads one into meditation."
(Bhagavad Gita)

Guidelines for Yoga Practice

General Guidelines

1. Wear loose, comfortable clothing and keep the feet bare. When you begin your yoga practice, close your eyes to check in with how you feel physically and emotionally. Let the breath relax and scan the body from head to toe and observe tight or tense areas. Then practice a few minutes of deep breathing (p. 47) to bring oxygen to the brain and relax the body.

2. The practice of a pose, or *asana*, is similar to climbing a ladder. Each step relates to a rung of a ladder. Do not try to climb beyond Level One of a pose if your body isn't strong in the lower stage. Maintaining body awareness as you move through each step will tell you whether or not you should go further.

3. While holding a pose, your focus on the breath as it sends energy through the body will keep the mind in touch with how the body feels. You will know if you need to ease up or come out of a pose, or if you can hold longer. Respect your body and stay in touch at *every* moment.

4. Be in touch with the quality of the breath while holding each pose. Breathe deeply and evenly. If breath becomes ragged or irregular, ease up. Breath helps you stay in touch with how far to climb up the ladder in your asana practice.

5. Move in and out of each pose slowly and carefully. When releasing, go back through each step in exactly the reverse order.

6. If a pose is too difficult to hold for long, come out of it slowly and try it again. This will help your body become familiar with what you are asking it to do, and the pose might be easier the second time. Whether or not you repeat a pose is up to you. In general, if you are able to hold the pose more than 30 seconds the first time, you do not need to repeat it. Repetition can help you build the strength to be able to hold a pose longer each time.

7. If you haven't time for a full workout or you have a headache or backache, find a pose to reach those areas where you are experiencing tension or discomfort (pp. 112–5).

Important Caveats

1. You should pay attention to several important caveats while doing yoga. First, in standing or seated poses where the legs are straight and tight, the kneecaps should be drawn up toward the hips, tightening the quadriceps. Be careful not to lock the knees. At the same time the quadriceps pull back toward the femur (thigh bone) to straighten the front of the leg and allow the back of the leg to release and stretch further.

2. Women in their moon cycle should rest when the flow is heavy and avoid any asana work. During the cycle, avoid inverted poses that hold the legs and pelvis above the head.

Alignment

Check the alignment of each part of the body while holding a pose. As you move further into the pose, do not lose the alignment you built on to get there.

While holding a pose and breathing deeply, be aware of the three main energy channels (*nadis*) of the torso: the center channel (*Sushumna*), the right channel (*Pingala*) and the left channel (*Ida*). For instance, in side bending, to keep these channels open and elongated, keep the chest forward and open, and in forward bending, keep the spine straight. Awareness of the nadis will help maintain proper alignment during a pose.

Be aware of the pelvic placement in each pose. In back-bending or standing poses, the tailbone drops down (slightly tucked). In forward bending (standing or seated), the pelvis tilts forward, releasing the tailbone.

To keep the spine straight in forward bends, visualize the alignment of each vertebra. Stack one on top of the other and feel each one separating to plump the disks (see diagram). You have seven cervical (neck) vertebrae, twelve thoracic (upper and mid-back) vertebrae, five lumbar (lower-back) vertebrae, four fused vertebrae in the sacrum (triangle bone) and two to four fused vertebrae in the coccyx (tailbone).

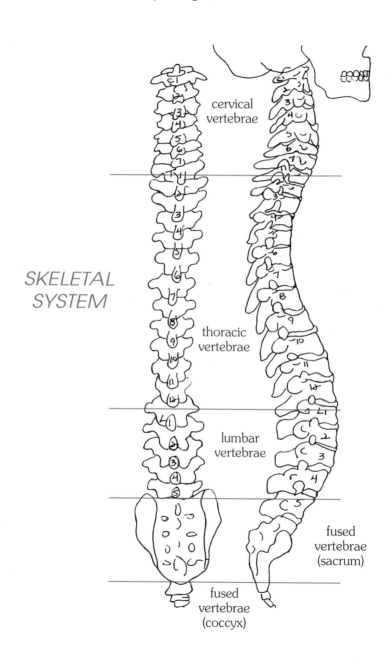

SKELETAL SYSTEM

cervical vertebrae

thoracic vertebrae

lumbar vertebrae

fused vertebrae (sacrum)

fused vertebrae (coccyx)

Holding Poses

A pose can be held as long as your body feels comfortable with it. Start with trying to hold 30 seconds and eventually build up to longer periods. When the lungs and body become stronger, the breathing deepens and you will be able to hold a pose longer.

Take time out to count your deep breaths against a clock for one minute. As you continue to practice, you will breathe fewer times in a minute because the lungs are clearer and able to fill deeper.

While holding a yoga pose, practice Ujjayi Breathing (Deep Breathing, p. 47).

Once you are familiar with practicing a particular asana, try to hold Mula Bandha (Root Lock, p. 99) while in the pose.

Your Individual Practice

Let your yoga practice be an intriguing, in-depth study of the internal and structural body, as you observe each breath you take and every move you make with conscious, inquisitive insight.

To set up a routine to practice on your own, pick a few poses from each category to stretch and strengthen every part of the body for a balanced workout. You should also practice by picking a pose that strengthens one area then immediately follow it with a counter-pose that stretches the same area out. Look in the back of this book for practice routines to follow (pp. 116–7).

Think of your yoga practice as your greatest teacher. It will balance the psyche and body, teaching you patience, humility, endurance, concentration, awareness, understanding, mental and physical strength, and flexibility. Enjoy this new awakening of the mind, body and spirit connecting with nature!

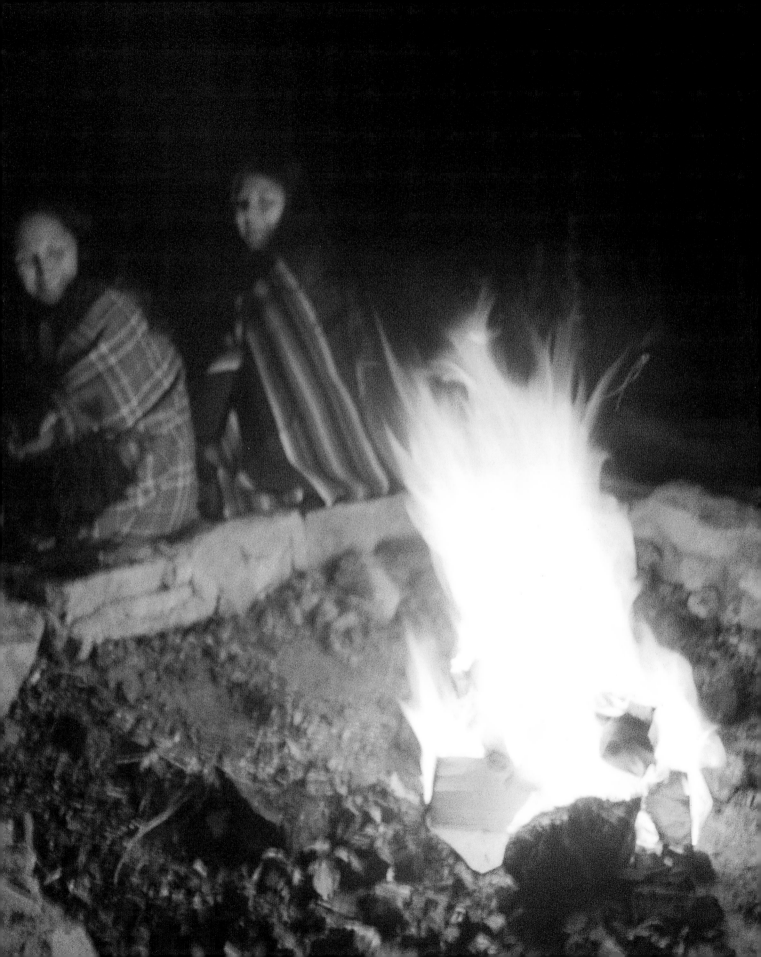

NATURE POSES

FIRE

Fire poses are used to produce heat and light in different areas of the body for inner strength and stability. Fire refers to the fire of digestion and elimination that re-creates the body every day and gives us vital energy. It also relates to light entering areas of the body that are heavy or blocked internally, such as the heart, throat or head. This light clears energy blocks.

Primary chakras involved with the Fire element
3rd chakra, Manipura, "lustrous gem"
7th chakra, Sahasrara, "thousandfold"

Fire Poses

"The raja yogi seeks nothing less than a complete transformation of self into a body of light."
(Patanjali, Yoga Sutras)

"This most excellent of asanas . . . makes the breath flow through the Sushumna, stimulates the gastric fire, makes the loins lean and removes all the diseases of men."
(Hatha Yoga Pradipika)

Shoulderstand Variations
(Sālamba Sarvāngāsana)

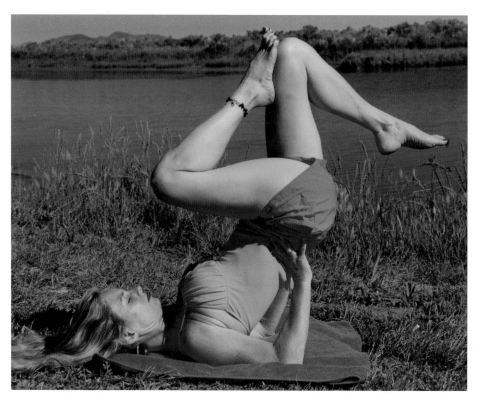

Variation I

- Start by lying down on the back with the arms resting to the sides of the body, legs straight.

- Take a deep breath and exhale to swing the legs and hips straight up in the air, supporting the hips with the hands. The spine angles back with the upper arms bearing the weight evenly from the shoulder to the elbow. Do not let the shoulders lift from the ground.

- If the neck hurts, fold a blanket and place it under the shoulders, so the neck has more space under it. In this case, the head rests lower than the shoulders.

- Once the back is supported by holding the hips, bend the right leg and place the foot on top of the left thigh near the knee. Then bend the left foot back toward the buttock.

- Hold as long as you feel strong in the pose, counting. Straighten both legs up to change sides. Hold the same amount of time on each side.

- Release by straightening the legs, bringing them overhead as far as you can to keep them close to the front of the body. Exhale and slowly lower the back down to the ground, one vertebra at a time, holding the legs up.

- When the back is relaxed down on the ground, the legs should be up at a right angle. Take a deep breath, flex both feet and slowly lower the legs straight down as you exhale.

- Bend the knees, wrap your arms around them and pull them to the chest. Relax.

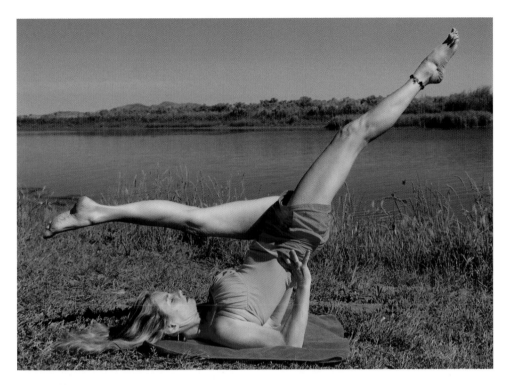

Variation II

- After following the steps in Variation I, you can try a different leg position in Shoulderstand. Straighten both legs up with the back angled, holding the hips. Take a deep breath, and on the exhalation split the legs open with the left leg overhead and the right leg back. Try to keep both legs straight.

- Hold as long as you feel strong in the pose, counting. Straighten both legs up and try splitting them the other way for the same amount of time.

- Release by straightening the legs, bringing them overhead as far as you can to keep them close to the front of the body. Exhale and slowly lower the back down to the ground, one vertebra at a time, holding the legs up.

- When the back is relaxed down on the ground, the legs should be up at a right angle. Take a deep breath, flex both feet and slowly lower the legs straight down as you exhale.

- Bend the knees, wrap your arms around them and pull them to the chest. Relax.

- You can practice Shoulderstand Variations Poses I and II separately, or let them flow one into the other after holding a good length of time on the first pose.

Benefits: Both of these poses build heat in the heart and upper body. They strengthen the back, buttocks, shoulders, arms, wrists and neck. They stretch the legs. They reverse the bloodflow and increase circulation throughout the body. Because these inverted positions bring a fresh supply of blood into the head, they clear the mind and are good for nonmigraine headaches and sinus problems. The pineal, pituitary, thyroid, thymus and adrenal glands, pancreas and gonads are stimulated.

Chakras: All the chakras are balanced.

Age level: Not suitable for ages 5 and under. Suitable for ages 6 and up.

Boat Pose
(Nāvāsana)

Benefits: This pose builds heat in the belly and hips. It strengthens the back, abdominal muscles, legs and hips. It tones the abdominal and reproductive organs. The nervous system and kidneys are stimulated. The pineal, pituitary, thyroid, thymus and adrenal glands, pancreas and gonads are stimulated.

Chakras: All the chakras are balanced.

Age level: Level One is suitable for ages 3 and up. Levels Two, Three and Four are suitable for ages 6 and up.

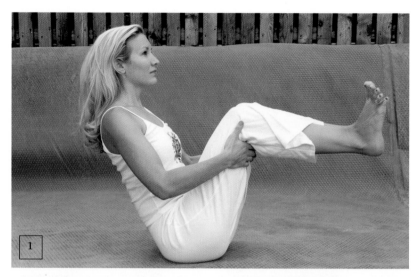

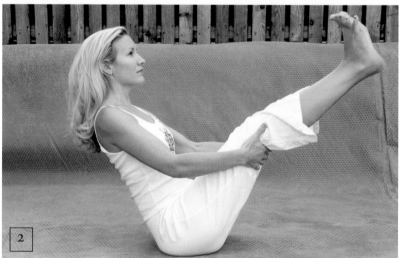

- Start in a seated position with the knees bent, placing the feet flat on the ground close to the buttocks. Hold the legs under the back of the knees.

- Lean back to balance on the tailbone with the spine straight and angled back (figure 1).

- *Level One:* Take a deep breath and exhale to lift the feet up to the height of the knees. Make sure the spine does not curve. Hold, breathing deeply, lifting the sternum with each inhalation to straighten the spine. Balance near the top of the sitbones (not on the lower back) and get grounded through the base of your body with your exhalations.

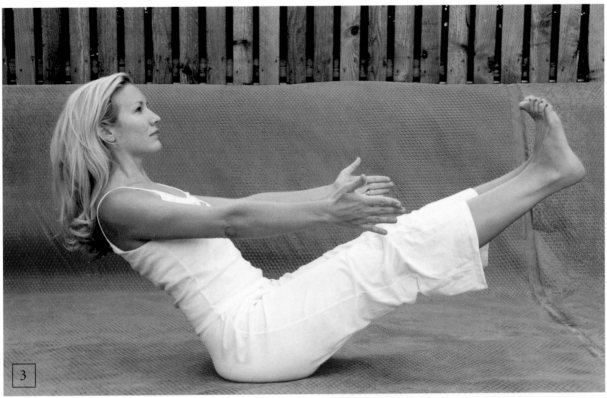

3

- *Level Two:* If the back is strong and held straight, you can try the next level. Exhale to straighten the legs and flex the feet. If the back begins to bend, hold the legs to pull the chest forward (figure 2).

- *Level Three:* If your back is strong and does not tend to bend, you can try the next level. (Otherwise, skip ahead to the last step.) Try to let go of the legs with the palms of the hands parallel to the outside of the knees. Focus upward on something to lift the chest, concentrate and balance (figure 3).

- *Level Four:* Once you are able to hold Level Three, you can try this next step. Hold onto the ankles or outer edges of the feet with both legs straight and use your exhalations to slowly draw them in toward the face (figure 4).

- Whichever level you are in, hold the pose, breathing deeply for one minute or more. To release, bend the knees and place the feet back on the ground. Rest the forehead on the knees and relax.

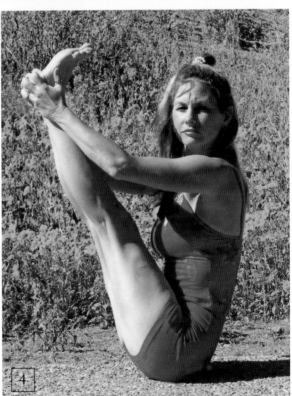

4

Partner Boat Pose
(Nāvāsana)

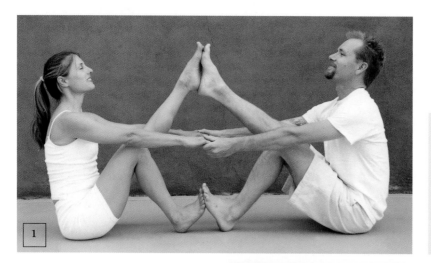

Benefits: This partner pose gives one all the benefits of Boat Pose along with added strength for the legs, since you can press against your partner's feet to keep the legs straight.

Chakras: All the chakras are balanced.

Age level: Suitable for ages 6 and up.

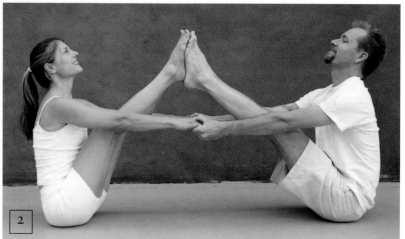

- Start in a seated position facing your partner with the legs bent, the feet close together on the ground.

- Extend the arms and hold each other's hands. Bend one leg and lift the foot up, pressing against your partner's foot to straighten the leg (figure 1). Now bend the other leg and lift the other foot up. Try to press against the other foot and raise it up until both legs are straight with the soles touching (figure 2).

- Lift the chest on each inhalation and exhale to check the balance through the base of the body.

- Hold, breathing deeply, fine-tuning the body positioning with each breath.

- Decide as partners when it is time to release, and go back through the steps in reverse to release the pose slowly.

- Relax with the forehead resting on the knees, legs bent.

Rolling Boat Pose
(Parivartanāsana Nāvāsana)

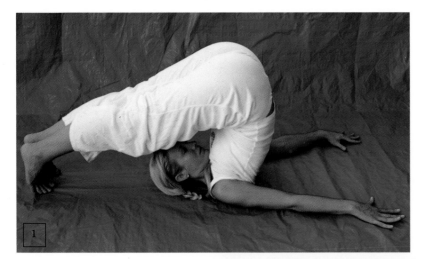

Benefits: This pose builds heat in the belly and lower body. It strengthens the back, hips, legs and abdominal muscles. It massages the spine, stimulating the nervous system and opening up blocked passageways to the brain. The pineal, pituitary, thyroid, thymus and adrenal glands, pancreas and gonads are stimulated.

Chakras: All the chakras are balanced.

Age level: Suitable for ages 6 and up.

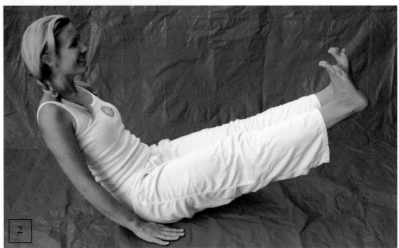

- Start in a seated position in Boat Pose (pp. 4–5).

- Place the hands on the ground beside the hips. Tuck the chin to the chest. Take a deep breath and exhale to roll back with the feet overhead (eventually bringing the toes to the ground), keeping the spine straight (figure 1).

- Take another deep breath and exhale to roll back up, balancing in Boat Pose, holding four deep breaths (figure 2). If the back and abdominal muscles are strong in Boat Pose, hold the back of the legs or ankles to roll back and up.

- Repeat the rolls five times. Then rest in a seated position with the knees bent, feet on the ground, forehead on the knees.

- Sit in Half or Full Lotus Pose (pp. 22–3) for a few moments to enjoy the tingling of the spine.

Revolved Head-to-Knee Pose
(Parivṛtta Jānu Sirṣāsana)

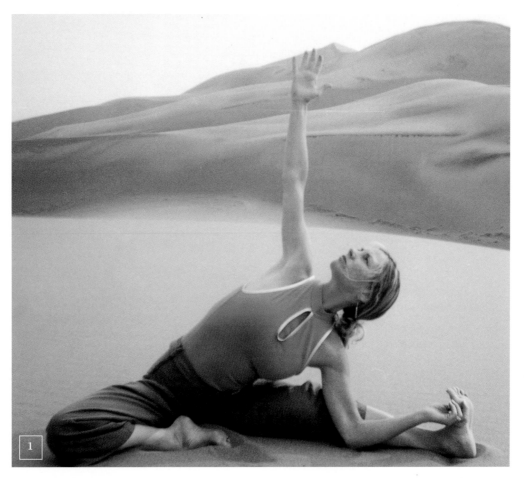

■ Start in a seated position with the soles of the feet together, heels close to the groin, knees open wide.

■ *Level One:* Take a deep breath, exhale to open the left leg out to the side as wide as you can without overstretching.

■ Keep the quadriceps tight and press the hamstrings down to the ground with the leg straight, foot flexed. The toes point directly up toward the sky.

■ Turn the top of the right foot down, allowing the heel to look up toward the sky.

■ Reach for the left foot or hold the left leg with the left hand. Inhale, raise the right arm up,

keeping the hand straight up from the shoulder, fingers wide. Look up to the hand. The chest is forward and open (figure 1).

■ Breathe deeply, lifting up through the waist and right arm on the inhalations, keeping the leg position strong on the exhalations, and slide down the left side over the leg.

■ *Level Two:* If the preceding level of the pose feels comfortable, exhale and reach the right arm overhead, with the elbow behind the ear. At this point you may be able to bring the left elbow down to the inside of the left knee, touching the ground and holding the instep of the left foot with the fingers, wrist turned up.

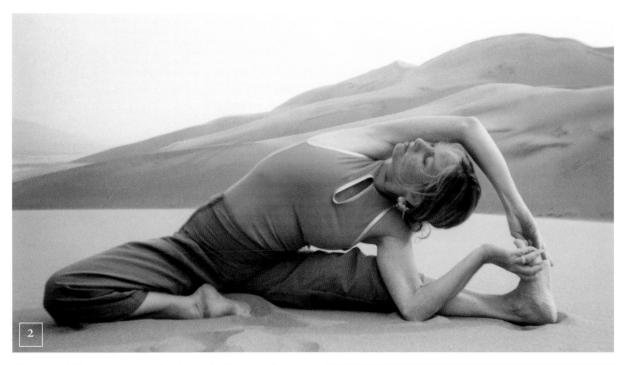

2

■ *Level Three:* Eventually the right hand will grasp the outside of the foot. Rotate the right ribs up toward the sky and breathe deeply through the right lung (figure 2).

■ Repeat to the other side.

Chakras: The 1st, 2nd, 3rd, 4th and 5th chakras are balanced.

Age level: Level One suitable for ages 3 and up. Levels Two and Three suitable for ages 6 and up.

Benefits: This pose builds heat in the center and lower body. It stretches the hamstrings on the outstretched leg, and the quadriceps. It stretches the hip flexors and front ankle on the bent leg. The waist, shoulders and arms are also stretching. It strengthens the back. The spleen and left kidney are stimulated when stretching over the left leg. When stretching to the right, the liver and kidney are stimulated. The digestive organs are stimulated. The thyroid, thymus and adrenal glands, pancreas and gonads are stimulated.

Rolling Bow Pose
(Dhanurāsana)

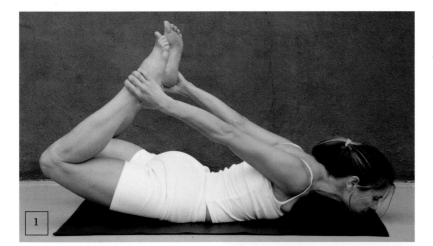

Chakras: The 1st, 2nd, 3rd, 4th and 5th chakras are balanced.

Age level: Suitable for ages 3 and up.

Benefits: This pose builds heat in the heart and belly. It massages the digestive organs and opens the front spine and chest, stretching the shoulders, arms and quadriceps. The thyroid, thymus and adrenal glands, pancreas and gonads are stimulated, along with the nervous system.

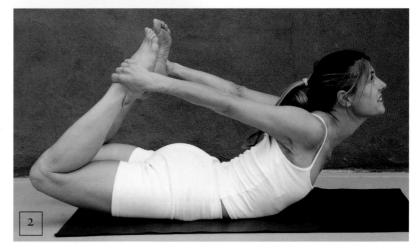

This pose is to be done on an empty stomach.

- Start lying face down, arms to the sides, chin on the ground.

- Bend the knees and flex the feet. Inhale to lift the chest up as high as you can, pressing the pelvis down,

with the tailbone tucked under and the buttocks tight. (This lengthens the lumbar vertebrae to protect the lower back.)

- Reach back with the chest lifted and hold the ankles. Take a deep breath, exhale and lift the thighs up from the ground. You are now in Bow Pose (figure 1).

- With the chest and thighs lifted, roll back and forth, massaging the front of the body (figure 2).

- Rolling as many times as you can, hold Bow Pose for five deep breaths and release the chest and arms first, then the legs. Relax in your starting position, turning the head to one side.

Navel Lock
(Uḍḍīyāna Bandha)

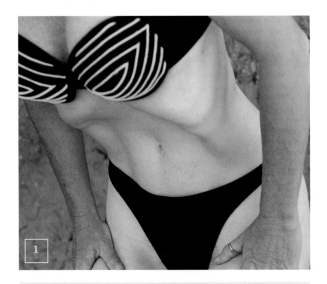

Benefits: This pose builds heat in the belly and is used for stimulating the peristaltic process for digestion. It strengthens the abdominal muscles and keeps the digestive organs cleansed. It is good for digestive problems such as constipation.

Chakras: The 3rd chakra is balanced.

Age level: Not suitable for ages 12 and under. Suitable for ages 13 and up.

To be done on an empty stomach.

■ Start in a standing position with the feet hip-width apart.

■ Place the hands on the thighs to push the skin down toward the knees. Lean forward slightly and take a breath, exhaling through the mouth.

■ After the air has emptied from the lungs fully, pull the abdominal muscles back toward the abdominal wall and up under the ribs. This creates a hollow space in the center of the belly (figure 1).

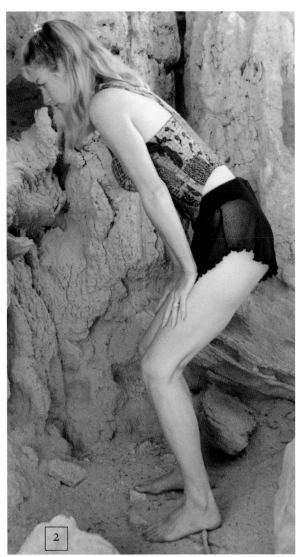

■ Hold as long as you can, counting (figure 2). Be careful not to strain. Holding without breath will be foreign to the body at first.

■ Release by taking a deep inhalation and exhaling through the nose. Repeat pose 5–10 times.

Supine Twist Pose
(Supta Parivartanāsana)

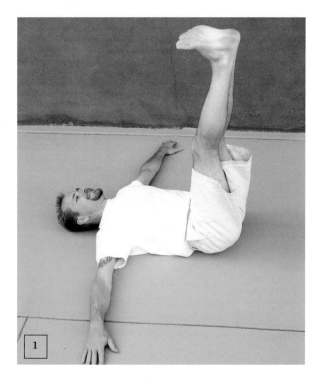

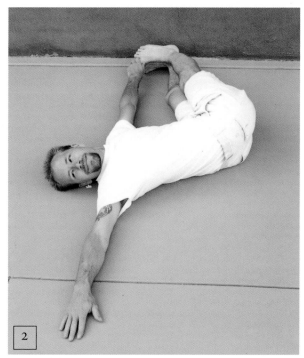

- Start lying down on the back with the legs straight on the ground. Extend the arms out across from the shoulders, palms down.

- Take a deep breath and exhale to lift both legs straight up to the sky, feet together and flexed. (If the back is tight, bend the knees into the chest then straighten them up.) Make sure the hips and shoulders are resting on the ground (figure 1).

- Take another deep breath, exhale and move both straight legs slowly to the left, toward the left hand on the ground. (If the back is tight, bend the knees to move the legs over to the left.)

- Look over the right shoulder. Breathe deeply and use the inhalations to stretch through the arms, keeping the shoulderblades down. On the exhalations, move the pelvis farther to the left, creating more twist in the spine. Flex both feet and push out through the heels (figure 2).

- Hold for one minute or more. Inhale to slowly lift both legs up toward the sky. Realign the spine on the ground before repeating to the other side. Hold the same length of time on the other side.

- To release, slowly lower both legs straight down, pressing out through the heels. Shake the legs out and relax.

Benefits: This pose builds heat in the belly and throat. The toning of the digestive organs helps digestive problems such as constipation. The spleen and liver are stimulated. The spine receives a fresh supply of blood to keep it healthy and to help open energy blocks to the brain. The thyroid, thymus and adrenal glands, pancreas and gonads are stimulated.

Chakras: The 1st, 2nd, 3rd, 4th and 5th chakras are balanced.

Age level: Suitable for ages 3 and up.

Seated V-Twist Pose
(Parivṛtta Upaviṣṭha Konāsana)

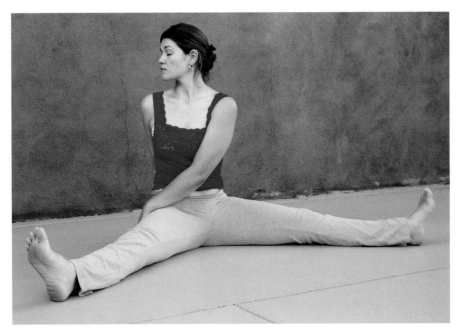

■ Start in a seated position with the legs open wide. Place the right hand behind the back on the ground near the tailbone, fingers pointing away from the body.

■ Keeping the spine straight, place the left hand on the outside of the right thigh. Take a deep breath and twist to the right on the exhalation.

Benefits: This pose builds heat in the belly, heart and throat. It stretches the chest, shoulders, hip flexors (adductors and psoas) and hamstrings. It strengthens the quadriceps, abdominal muscles, back and lungs. The digestive organs, spinal column, heart, spleen and liver are stimulated. The thyroid, thymus and adrenal glands, pancreas and gonads are stimulated.

■ Breathe deeply, lifting the sternum on the inhalations and twisting farther on the exhalations. Look over the right shoulder and open it when twisting. Let the hips move to the right with the chest, but keep the sitbones on the ground.

■ Hold for one minute or more. Release slowly and repeat to the other side for the same amount of time.

Chakras: The 1st, 2nd, 3rd, 4th and 5th chakras are balanced.

Age level: Suitable for ages 3 and up.

Standing Backbend Pose
(Ūrdhva Dhanurāsana Prep)

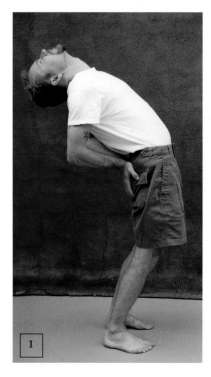

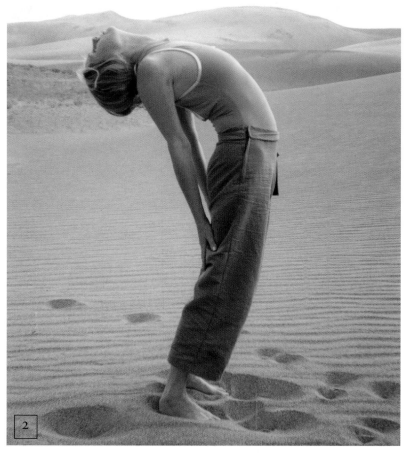

Chakras: All the chakras are balanced.

Age level: Suitable for ages 3 and up.

■ Stand with the feet hip-width apart, toes wide and directly forward. Keep the legs tight and drop the tailbone down.

■ *Level One:* Place the hands against the buttocks and press downward. Inhale and stretch back to open the chest holding the shoulders away from the ears, squeezing the shoulderblades together. Hold the pose for one minute or more, breathing deeply (figure 1).

■ *Level Two:* Eventually walk the hands down the back of the thighs to create more bend in the back. Focus on stretching from the pubic bone back through the crown of the head, opening the front of the spine (figure 2).

■ Inhale to release, standing straight, then exhale to rest the arms to the sides. Relax in a standing position.

Benefits: This pose builds heat in the lower back. It stretches the front of the spine, abdominal muscles, chest, shoulders and throat. It strengthens the legs, ankles and back. The kidneys, spleen and nervous system are stimulated. The pineal, pituitary, thyroid, thymus and adrenal glands, pancreas and gonads are stimulated.

Half Camel Variation Pose
(Ardha Ūṣṭrāsana)

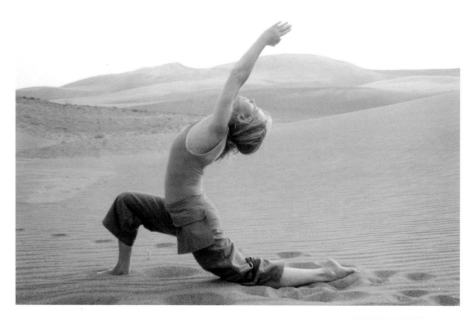

- Start on the hands and knees with the hands under the shoulders, palms flat, fingers pointing straight forward and wide. The knees are hip-width apart directly under the hips, with the spine long.

- Place the right foot flat on the ground between the hands, with the knee over the heel to create a right angle.

- Slide the left leg straight back with the knee, shin and front of the ankle on the ground and the big toe pointing straight back.

- Inhale and reach the arms overhead with the palms together, elbows back behind the ears.

- Look up at the fingers. On the inhalation, stretch up to straighten the arms. Exhale to drop the hips down and even the weight out through both legs, bending the back.

- Hold for one minute or more, breathing deeply, concentrating on trying to bend back farther.

- To release, inhale and straighten the spine, looking forward. Exhale to release the arms to the sides with the palms beside the right foot. Slide the right leg back to your starting position on the hands and knees.

- Repeat to the other side for the same amount of time.

- When finished with both sides, sit back on the heels with the arms to the sides, forehead down on the ground (Child's Pose, pp. 58–9) and rest for a moment.

Benefits: This pose builds heat in the lower back. It stretches the leg that is extended back, along with the hip flexors, chest and arms. It strengthens the back, hips and legs. The kidneys and spleen are stimulated. The pineal, pituitary, thyroid, thymus and adrenal glands, pancreas and gonads are stimulated.

Chakras: All the chakras are balanced.

Age level: Not suitable for ages 5 and under. Suitable for ages 6 and up.

Balance-on-Wall—Forward Bend Pose
(Utthiṭa Hasta Pādanguṣṭhāsana Variation)

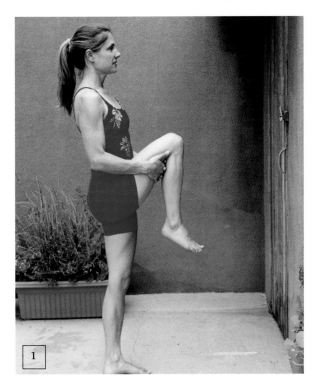

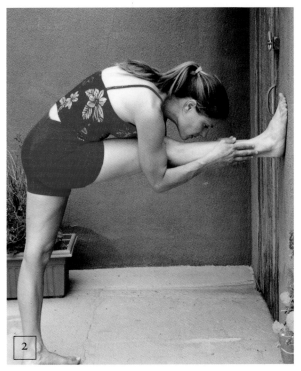

■ Stand facing a wall, approximately 3 feet away from it, with the feet together. Bend the right leg and hold under the bent knee to balance on the left foot. Drop the tailbone and keep the left leg tight (figure 1).

■ Place the right foot straight across from the hip into the wall, toes pointing up.

■ *Level One:* Inhale to raise the arms overhead, then exhale to move the torso forward and reach along the leg toward the wall. Take a few deep breaths to lengthen the spine and move the abdomen and then the chest down over the front thigh.

■ *Level Two:* Eventually bring the head down to the shin (figure 2). Do not bend at the center of the back. If the hips or hamstrings are tight, stay up higher with the hands above the foot until you can come into a full forward bend with the front of the body resting on the front leg.

■ Hold for one minute or more, breathing deeply. Inhale to lengthen the spine; exhale to move forward.

■ To release, inhale and lift the torso up, then exhale to release the leg from the wall, supporting the back of the knee with the hands.

■ Repeat to the other side for the same amount of time.

Benefits: This pose builds heat in the abdomen. It strengthens the standing leg, hip and ankle. The hamstrings are stretched on both legs. During forward bending, the blood is moving forward to tone the digestive organs. The pineal, pituitary, thyroid, thymus and adrenal glands, pancreas and gonads are stimulated.

Chakras: All the chakras are balanced.

Age level: Not suitable for ages 5 and under. Suitable for ages 6 and up.

Balance-on-Wall—Twist Pose
(*Parivṛtta Hasta Pādanguṣṭhāsana* Variation)

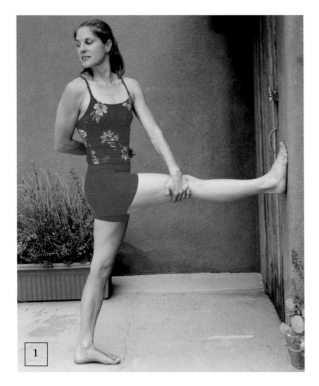

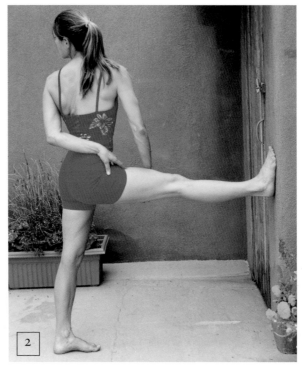

This pose can be done as a continuation of Balance-on-Wall—Forward Bend Pose, or you may go back through the opening stages of that pose before moving on to this twist.

- With the right leg up on the wall, keep the spine straight and both legs tight. Place the left hand on the outside of the right leg near the knee. Reach around the back, placing the right hand on the waist, or hold the inner thigh of the left leg if you can.

- Take a deep breath and twist to the right on the exhalation. Hold breathing deeply.

- Lift the sternum up on the inhalation, twisting farther on the exhalation. Feel the energy working through both legs to keep them strong (figure 1).

- Hold for one minute or more and untwist. Repeat the twist to the other side, holding for the same amount of time (figure 2).

- Release the right leg by holding under the back knee. Take a deep breath, standing on both feet.

- Now repeat by lifting the left leg and holding the twists to both sides.

Benefits: This pose builds heat in the belly and throat. It strengthens the abdominal muscles along with the standing leg, hip and ankle. The spinal twist adds more stimulation to the digestive organs and keeps the spine flexible, massaging the nerves and stimulating the brain. The pineal, pituitary, thyroid, thymus and adrenal glands, pancreas and gonads are stimulated.

Chakras: All the chakras are balanced.

Age level: Not suitable for ages 5 and under. Suitable for ages 6 and up.

Cow Twist Pose
(Parivṛtta Gomukāsana)

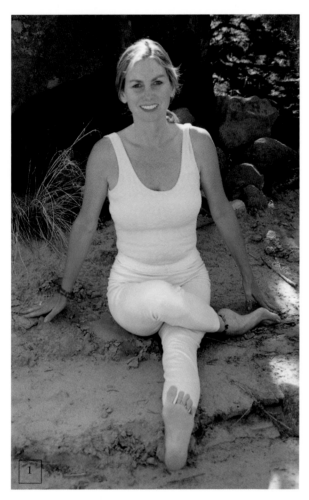

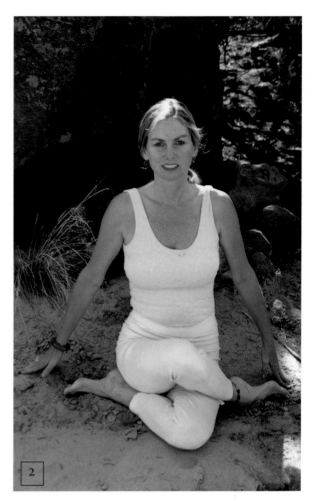

- Start in a seated position with the legs straight out in front of the body.

- *Level One:* Cross the right leg over the left with the right knee directly over the left knee. The top of the right foot rests on the ground with the toes pointing back. Keep both sitbones evenly on the ground (figure 1).

- If the hips are tight, stay at this stage to work on the spinal twist with the left leg straight out in front. Skip ahead to the instructions at the top left column of the next page.

- *Level Two:* Bend the left leg back, bringing the foot close to the right buttock (figure 2).

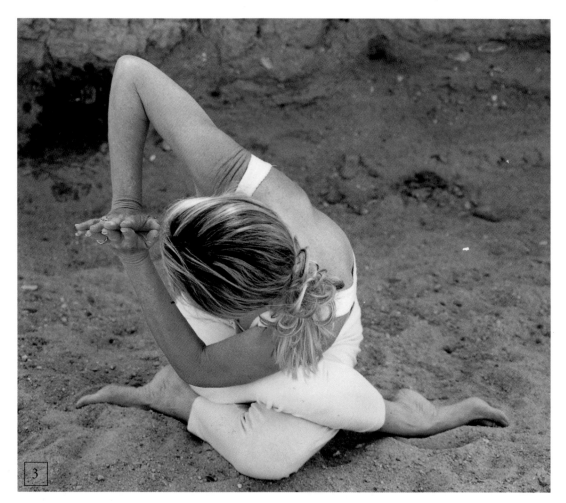

3

- From the leg position of either Level One or Level Two, stretch forward and hook the left elbow around to the outside of the right knee, as low as you can. Place the palms together and begin the spinal twist by raising the right elbow up as high as you can to open the chest (figure 3).

- Hold for one minute or more, breathing deeply and twisting farther on the exhalations.

- Release the twist of the spine and stretch forward over the knees to lengthen the back. Inhale, lift the torso up slowly, straighten the spine and release the left leg first, then the right. Shake the legs out.

- Repeat to the other side, holding for the same amount of time.

Benefits: This pose stretches the chest, shoulders, hips, hip flexors, quadriceps and ankles. The spinal twist strengthens the back and abdominal muscles. The heart, digestive organs, lungs, spleen, liver and nervous system are stimulated. The pineal, pituitary, thyroid, thymus and adrenal glands, pancreas and gonads are stimulated.

Chakras: All the chakras are balanced.

Age level: Not suitable for ages 5 and under. Suitable for ages 6 and up.

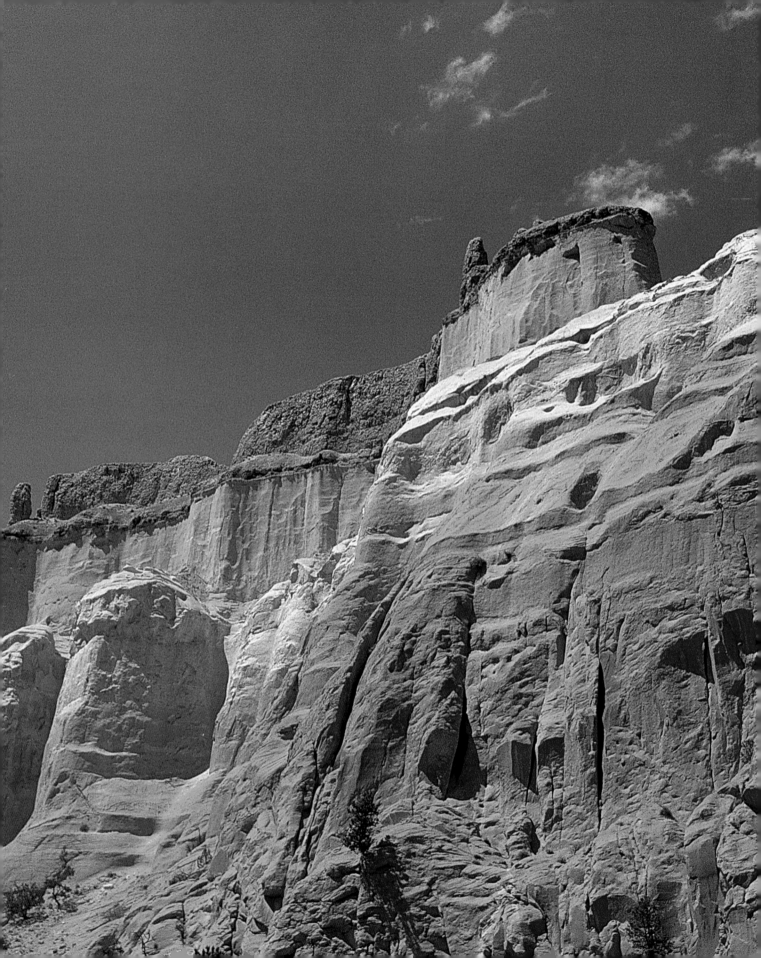

EARTH

Earth poses relate to the most solid parts of our body and the way we are affected by gravity. Grounding energy is brought downward through different parts of the body when connecting to the Earth—the feet, buttocks, hands or head.

Primary chakras involved with Earth element
1st chakra, Muladhara, "root"
7th chakra, Sahasrara, "thousandfold"

Earth Poses

"Yoga pose is mastered by relaxation of effort, lessening the tendency for restless breathing, and promoting an identification of oneself as living within the infinite breath of life."
(Patanjali, Yoga Sutras)

"From that perfection of Yoga posture, duality, such as reacting to praise and criticism, ceases to be a disturbance."
(Patanjali, Yoga Sutras)

Half Lotus Pose
(Ardha Pādmāsana)

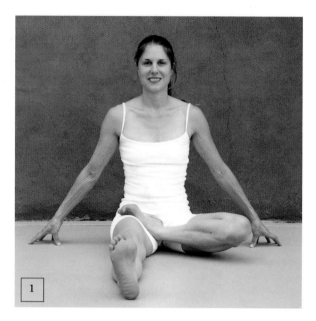

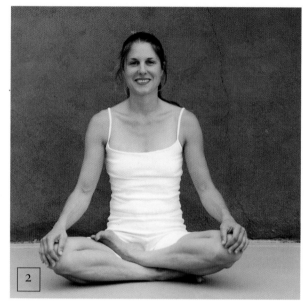

- Start in a seated position with the legs straight out in front, spine straight.

- *Level One:* Cross the left leg over the right with the top of the left foot resting on top of the right thigh, toes pointing back (figure 1). If the hips are too tight, continue the steps of this pose, but do not use the leg position of Level Two. Instead, keep the right leg straight out. Place the hands on the knees with the thumbs and index fingers touching. Relax the shoulders down from the ears and open the chest.

Benefits: This pose brings the energy down into the lower body to connect with the Earth. It stretches the hips and ankles. It opens the chest and lungs to bring more oxygen to the brain. It strengthens the back muscles. The reproductive organs are toned, and the nervous system is stimulated. The pineal, pituitary, thyroid, thymus and adrenal glands, pancreas and gonads are stimulated.

- *Level Two:* Bend the right leg under the left (figure 2).

- Using the leg position of either Level One or Level Two, breathe deeply and focus on the inhalations spiraling the energy up the spine to lift the crown of the head. Let the exhalations spiral down the spine to drop down the tailbone, keeping the sitbones even. If you can, press the knees down toward the ground. Hold for one minute or more.

- To release, straighten the right and then the left leg out in front.

- Repeat to the other side. Hold for the same amount of time, then release.

- Shake the legs out and roll the feet in circles to stretch out the ankles.

Chakras: All the chakras are balanced in this pose, especially the 1st and 2nd.

Age level: Suitable for ages 3 and up.

Full Lotus Pose
(Pādmāsana)

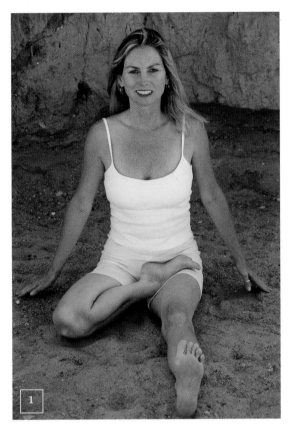

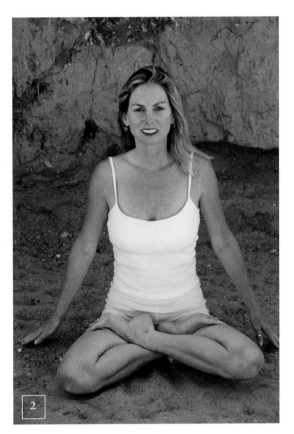

Practice this once the Half Lotus Pose (opposite page) feels comfortable with the knees pressed down toward the ground.

▦ Start in a seated position with the legs straight out in front, spine straight.

▦ Cross the right leg over the left with the top of the right foot resting on top of the left thigh, toes pointing back (figure 1).

▦ If the right knee is down toward the ground, you can move on to complete the Full Lotus. Otherwise, keep working in Half Lotus Pose until the hips open more.

Benefits: This pose gives the same benefits as the Half Lotus Pose, with added stretch for the ankles and hips.

▦ Keeping the right knee down toward the ground, cross the left leg over the right, with the top of the left foot resting on top of the right thigh, toes pointing back. The heels will point toward the navel (figure 2).

▦ Hold for one minute or more, breathing deeply and focusing on the energy spiraling up and down the spine.

▦ Release the left leg first and then the right. Shake the legs out and roll the feet in circles to stretch the ankles.

▦ Repeat to the other side, noticing if one hip is tighter than the other.

Chakras: All the chakras are balanced, especially the 1st and 2nd.

Age level: Not suitable for ages 5 and under. Suitable for ages 6 and up.

Lotus Lift Pose
(*Utthiṭa Pādmāsana*)

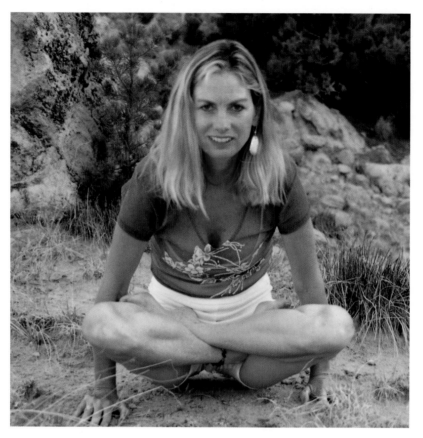

- Start in either Half or Full Lotus Pose (pp. 22–3).

- Place the hands in front of the hips, palms flat on the ground, fingers wide, pointing straight ahead.

- Push down through the hands and exhale to lift the buttocks off the ground. (If you are not able to work in Full Lotus Pose and you are in Half Lotus Pose, the bottom leg will stay on the ground, but you can still lift the buttocks.)

Benefits: This pose requires a lot of strength and connects the hands into the Earth for grounding. It gives the same benefits as Half or Full Lotus Pose with added strength for the heart, wrists, arms, shoulders and abdominal muscles.

- Hold as long as you can, then release the buttocks down to the ground gently. Sit with the spine straight and take a deep breath.

- Release the legs and repeat to the other side and lift. Hold for the same amount of time.

- Shake the legs out and roll the feet in circles.

Chakras: All the chakras are balanced.

Age level: Not suitable for ages 5 and under. Suitable for ages 6 and up.

Blossoming Flower (group pose)
(Supta Konāsana)

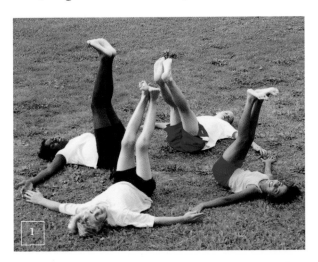

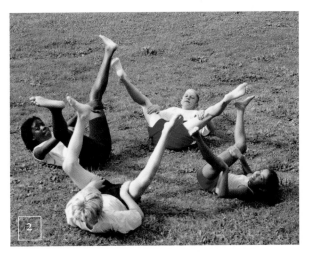

This pose can be done with three or more people.

- Start lying on the back in a circle with the legs straight, feet touching in the center. Reach your arms out across from the shoulders, touching your partners' hands on either side.

- Take a deep breath and exhale to lift both legs straight up toward the sky, feet flexed. Keeping the back on the ground, breathe deeply, trying to push up through the heels and tighten the front of the legs. Hold this position for five deep breaths (figure 1).

- Take a deep breath and exhale to open both legs evenly, as wide as you can. Hold the inner thighs and straighten the legs. Hold this position, breathing deeply, keeping the back on the ground, trying to widen the legs more as you exhale.

Chakras: The 1st, 2nd, 3rd, 4th and 5th chakras are balanced.

Age level: Suitable for ages 3 and up.

- After holding with the back down for at least five deep breaths, exhale and lift the chest and head up to look through the legs. Hold this position for five deep breaths (figure 2).

- To release, exhale and roll the back and head down.

- Then inhale to bring the legs together toward the sky. Keep the legs straight, feet flexed.

- Take a deep breath and exhale to slowly lower the legs straight down. Shake the legs out and relax with the arms to the sides of the body.

Benefits: This group pose brings the energy down through the back to connect to the Earth. It strengthens the neck, back, abdominal muscles and front of the legs. It stretches the shoulders, arms, upper back, hips and hip flexors, and the back of the legs. The liver, gall bladder, spleen, and digestive and abdominal organs are toned. The thyroid, thymus and adrenal glands, pancreas and gonads are stimulated.

Tree in Half Lotus Pose
(Vṛkṣāsana)

If you have a hard time with balance, stand with your back against a wall to support the body.

- Start in a standing position with the feet together, toes wide, heels open slightly. Both feet are aligned directly forward. The arms rest at the sides of the body with the shoulders dropped down away from the ears and the chest open. Take a few deep breaths and send the energy down through the feet. Keep the legs tight, getting grounded. The tailbone drops down. You are now in Mountain Pose.

- Focus on a spot in front and exhale to lift the right foot and place it on top of the left thigh in a Half Lotus position (p. 22).

- Once you are balanced and grounded on the left foot, place the hands in prayer position to the heart center. The thumbs touch the thymus (Anjali Mudra, figure 1).

- Hold for one minute or more, breathing deeply. Focus on the inhalations moving energy up through the crown of the head and the exhalations sending energy down through the left foot into the Earth.

- To release, bring the arms down first, then hold the right foot to place it down on the ground. Take a deep breath in Mountain Pose to get grounded through both feet.

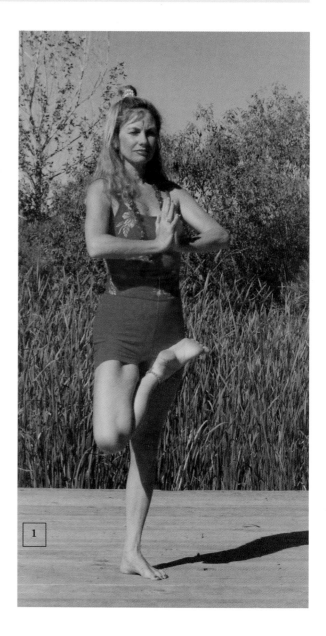

1

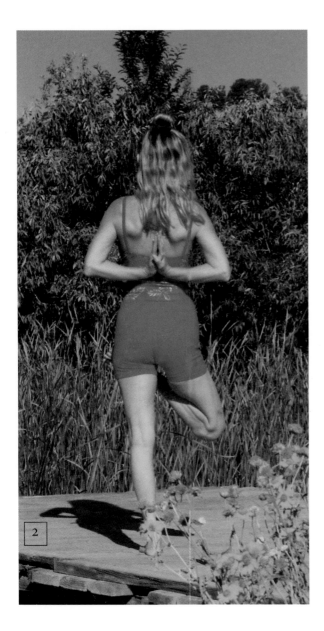

2

■ Repeat to the other side and hold for the same amount of time. When finished, take a few deep breaths in Mountain Pose and observe the heaviness created through the base of the body.

■ *Variation:* If you are able to hold strong in this pose, try a variation. Place the hands behind the back in prayer position (figure 2). If that is too difficult, clasp the elbows behind the back to open the chest.

Benefits: This pose brings energy down through the feet to connect to the Earth. It strengthens the back, hips, legs and ankles. The wrists are stretched. It is a balance pose that develops concentration and strengthens the mind. The pineal, pituitary, thyroid, thymus and adrenal glands, pancreas and gonads are stimulated.

Chakras: All the chakras are balanced.

Age level: Not suitable for ages 5 and under. Suitable for ages 6 and up.

Tree in Half Lotus Wrap Pose
(Ardha Baddha Pādmottanāsana)

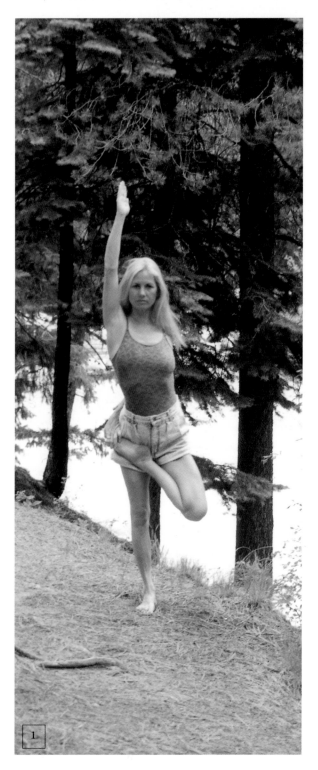

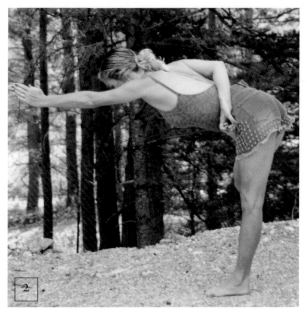

If you have a hard time with balance, stand with the right side of the body near a wall and hold the wall with the right hand. Stand with the left side near the wall when you repeat the pose on the other side.

■ Start in a standing position with the feet together, toes wide, heels open slightly. Both feet are aligned directly forward. The arms rest at the sides of the body with the shoulders dropped down away from the ears and the chest open. Take a few deep breaths and send the energy down through the feet. Keep the legs tight, getting grounded. The tailbone drops down (Mountain Pose, p. 26).

■ Focus on a spot in front and exhale to lift the right foot and place it on top of the left thigh in a Half Lotus position (p. 22).

■ *Level One:* Once you are balanced and grounded through the right foot, reach the left arm around the back of the waist and hold onto the big toe of the left foot. If the shoulders are tight and you can't reach the foot, put a strap around the top of the foot and hold the strap. The chest stays forward and open.

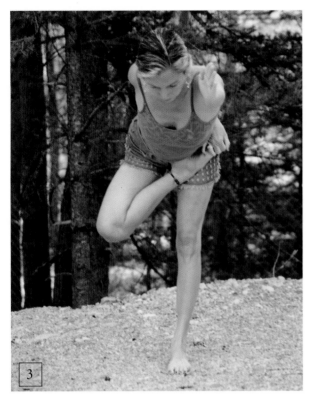

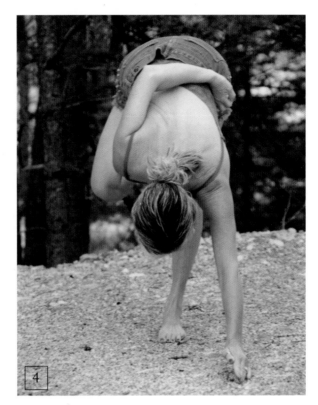

- Inhale and raise the right arm, keeping the elbow close to the side of the head.

- Hold for one minute or more, breathing deeply. Concentrate and focus on the inhalations stretching up through the right hand. The exhalations bring the energy down through the right foot. Feel the openness through the belly (figure 1).

- To release, lower the right arm to the side of the body, let go of the left foot and bring the left arm and left foot down. Stand in Mountain Pose and take a deep breath.

- Repeat to the other side.

- *Level Two:* If you feel strong in this pose, try a forward bend. Focus on a spot in front and exhale to bring the torso down into a tabletop position with the spine straight, the elbow close to the head and the right arm extended out (figures 2 and 3).

Chakras: All the chakras are balanced.

Age level: Not suitable for ages 12 and under. Suitable for ages 13 and up.

- *Level Three:* If the hamstrings will allow you to go farther, let the torso move forward until you can reach for the ground with the right hand. Your focal point will move in toward the right foot as you bring the torso down (figure 4). Hold for a few breaths, then inhale to lift the spine straight up. Take a deep breath.

- To release, lower the right arm down to the side of the body, let go of the left foot and bring the left arm and foot down. Stand in Mountain Pose and take a deep breath.

- Repeat to the other side.

Benefits: This pose brings the energy down through the feet to connect to the Earth. It strengthens the hip, leg and ankle of the standing leg. It stretches the hip flexors and the hip and ankle of the bent leg. It stretches the shoulders and opens the chest. Balancing on one leg develops concentration to strengthen the mind. The pineal, pituitary, thyroid, thymus and adrenal glands, pancreas and gonads are stimulated.

Tree in Open Leg Twist Pose
(Parivṛtta Utthiṭa Pādanguṣṭhāsana)

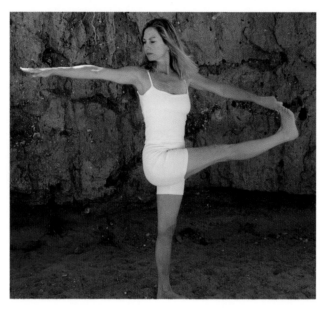

Start in a standing position in Mountain Pose (p. 26). Take a few deep breaths and send the energy down through the feet with the legs tight, getting grounded. The tailbone drops down.

Focus on a spot in front and inhale to bring the arms out across from the shoulders. Exhale to bend the right leg into the chest, holding onto the big toe with the left hand (middle finger, index finger and thumb). Balancing, keep the left leg tight. Take another deep breath and exhale to straighten the right leg out in front of the body with the foot across from the right hip. If the hamstrings are too tight, keep the knee bent or use a strap around your foot to keep your leg straight.

If you have a difficult time balancing, stand with the right side of the body near a wall and hold the wall with the right arm extended beyond the right shoulder to open the chest.

Otherwise, hold onto the big toe and twist the spine with the right arm extended out, and look over the right shoulder.

Chakras: All the chakras are balanced.

Age level: Not suitable for ages 12 and under. Suitable for ages 13 and up.

Hold for one minute or more, breathing deeply. Inhale to lift the spine, then exhale to stay grounded and press down through the right heel. Continue opening the chest and twist farther.

To release, untwist, bend the right leg into the chest and bring it down to the ground. Take a deep breath in Mountain Pose.

Repeat to the other side and hold for the same amount of time. If using a wall to balance, turn the left side of the body toward the wall and hold it with the left hand.

Benefits: This pose brings the energy down through the feet to connect to the Earth. It strengthens the back, hips, abdominal muscles, legs and ankles. It stretches the shoulders, chest, arms and neck. Balancing on one leg develops concentration. The spinal twist opens energy blocks through the spine to stimulate the brain and digestive organs. The spleen, liver, gall bladder and kidneys are stimulated. The pineal, pituitary, thyroid, thymus and adrenal glands, pancreas and gonads are stimulated.

Forest Trees (group pose)
(Vṛkṣāsana)

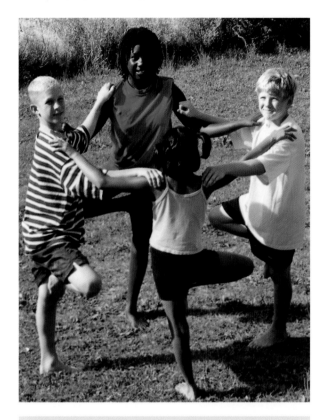

Benefits: *This group pose brings the energy down through the feet to connect to the Earth. It strengthens the standing hip, leg and ankle along with the abdominal muscles. The chest is opened and shoulders and hip flexors are stretched. The lymph nodes on the inner thigh near the groin are stimulated when the leg is bent, and the sole of the foot pushes into the thigh. The pineal, pituitary, thyroid, thymus and adrenal glands, pancreas and gonads are stimulated.*

Chakras: All the chakras are balanced.

Age level: Suitable for ages 3 and up.

- With a group of three or more, start in a standing position in a circle facing one another, slightly less than one arm length apart. Stand with feet together in Mountain Pose (p. 26) and take a deep breath. Raise the right foot and place it on the inside of the left thigh with the heel near the groin. Press the knee down toward the ground, opening the knee wide, and push the sole of the foot against the inner thigh.

- Balance and keep the left leg tight, dropping the tailbone.

- Inhale to reach your arms out to hold onto your partners' shoulders on both sides of you.

- Hold for one minute or more, breathing deeply. Inhale to lift the chest up and exhale, opening the right knee out and pressing down through the left foot. Concentrate and focus on balancing alone. Be careful not to count on your partners to hold you up.

- Decide as a group when it is time to release. Take the arms down to the sides of the body and release the right leg.

- Take a deep breath with the feet together in Mountain Pose. Repeat to the other side, holding for the same amount of time.

Tripod Pose
(Sirṣāsana Prep)

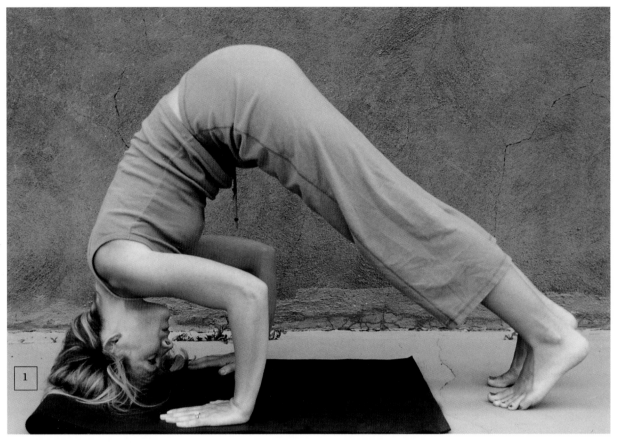

- Start on the hands and knees. Place the palms flat on the ground, shoulder-width apart, fingers wide and pointing directly forward.

- *Level One:* Put the crown of the head on the ground in front of the hands, creating a triangle position from the head to the hands. Curl the toes under.

- Take a deep breath and exhale to raise the knees from the ground and straighten the legs.

- If the neck is weak and it is uncomfortable to rest more weight on the crown of the head, stay in this beginning stage of the pose to strengthen the neck. The weight is held even through the head and the hands. Lift the shoulders toward the sky to lengthen the neck (figure 1).

- *Level Two:* Keeping weight on the crown of the head, begin walking the feet in toward the face to lift the tailbone up and straighten the spine.

- Bend one leg and place the shin on top of the upper arm with the knee near the armpit. Practice holding one leg up at a time.

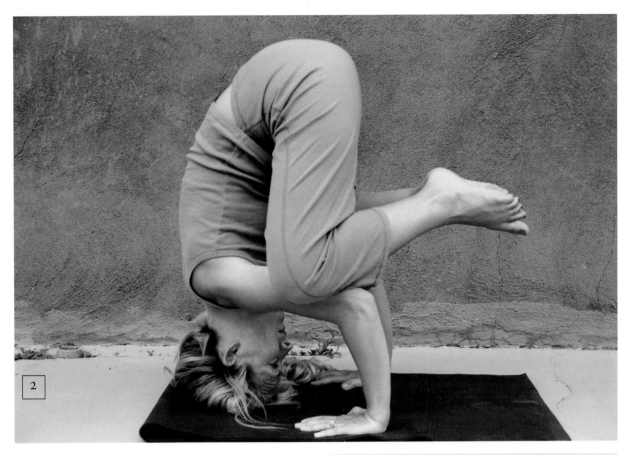

2

■ *Level Three:* When you feel strong enough, bring both legs up on the upper arms. Once both legs are resting on the arms, bring the toes together, with the back straight (figure 2).

■ Tighten the anal sphincter (Mula Bandha, p. 99) and hold Navel Lock (Uddiyana Bandha, p. 11) while staying in this pose.

■ Hold for one minute or more, breathing deeply. Lift the shoulders and tailbone toward the sky on the inhalations. Focus on pressing down through the hands and head with the exhalations.

■ To release, take one leg down at a time, then walk the feet away from the face. Rest by sitting back on the heels, forehead down, arms resting to the sides (Child's Pose, pp. 58–9). Relax!

Benefits: This pose brings the energy down through the head and hands to connect to the Earth. It strengthens the neck, back, shoulders, arms, heart, abdominal muscles and wrists. The blood moving into the head relieves headaches and clears the mind. It stretches the hips and back. The abdominal organs and digestive organs are massaged and toned. The pineal, pituitary, thyroid, thymus and adrenal glands, pancreas and gonads are stimulated.

Chakras: All the chakras are balanced, especially the 7th.

Age level: Not suitable for ages 5 and under. Suitable for ages 6 and up.

Headstand Pose
(Sirṣāsana)

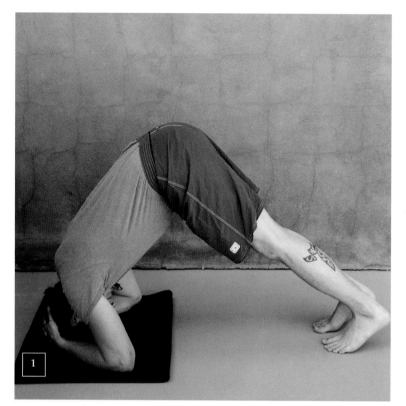
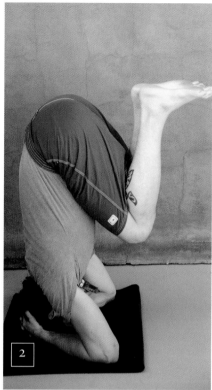

This pose can be practiced with the back against a wall or in a corner of two walls until you are strong enough to balance on your own.

- Start on the hands and knees. Interlock the fingers, with the forearms down on the ground and elbows under the shoulders. The palms are open to make a cup.

- Place the crown of the head on the ground, holding the back of the head with the fingers and open palms. Keep the wristbones toward the sky so the wrists don't fall open. This prevents stress on the wrists once the body is fully lifted.

- *Level One:* Take a deep breath and exhale to curl the toes under and lift the knees up to straighten the legs (figure 1). If the neck feels weak, hold at this level, lifting the tailbone toward the sky and pushing down through the heels to stretch the backs of the legs.

- *Level Two:* If the neck feels strong, begin walking the feet in toward the face. Make sure the hands and forearms press down and you stay on the crown of the head. Lift the feet off the ground and tuck the knees into the chest, straightening the spine (figure 2).

- Slowly straighten the legs up and lift through the balls of the feet with the legs together, rolling them toward each other from the groin.

- Eventually the body is lifted in a vertical line with the feet straight up from the hips. Pull the front ribs and abdominal muscles back toward the backside. Lift the tailbone up with a slight tuck and keep the buttocks strong (figure 3).

- Hold for one minute or more, breathing deeply. Inhale to lift the shoulders, spine and legs. Exhale to focus on getting balanced evenly through both forearms and the crown of the head.

- Once you are comfortable doing Headstand, practice tightening the anal sphincter (Mula Bandha, p. 99) and the Navel Lock (Uddiyana Bandha, p. 11) while holding the pose.

- To release, bend the knees into the chest and slowly lower the legs. Walk the feet away from the face and sit back on the heels, forehead down, arms resting to the sides (Child's Pose, pp. 58–9). Relax!

Benefits: This pose increases circulation through the entire body and is considered to be the "King" or "Father" of all asanas. You are solid like a mountain in a reverse position. Headstand brings the energy down through the head and forearms to connect to the Earth. It reverses the blood flow into the heart and head, stimulating the mind and strengthening the lungs and heart. The neck, back, arms, wrists and abdominal muscles are strengthened. The abdominal organs, liver and spleen are bathed in blood for stimulation. The pineal, pituitary, thyroid, thymus and adrenal glands, pancreas and gonads are stimulated.

Chakras: All the chakras are balanced, especially the 7th.

Age level: Level One suitable for ages 3–12. Other levels suitable for ages 13 and up.

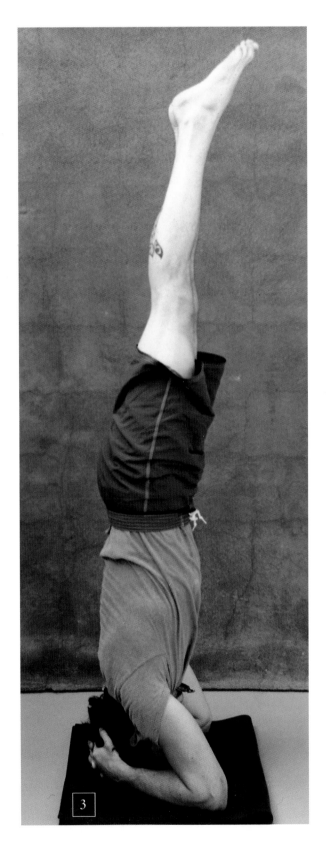

3

Standing Vine Pose
(Ūrdhva Parivṛtta Hastāsana)

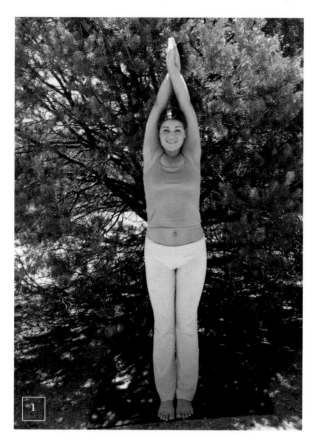

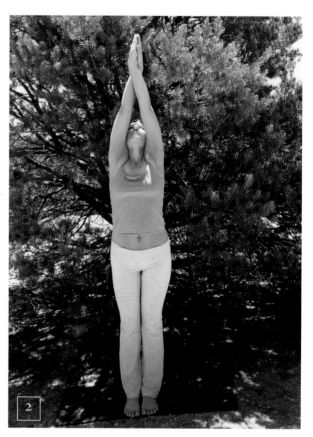

- Start in a standing position with the feet together in Mountain Pose (p. 26).

- Inhale to raise the arms up overhead, crossing the wrists and turning the upper arms in toward each other, palms together. Keep the arms straight with the elbows back behind the ears (figure 1).

- Breathe deeply for five breaths, reaching up through the arms with the inhalations. Use the exhalations to move the elbows back behind the ears and drop the shoulders down, getting grounded through the feet.

- Take a deep breath and exhale to bring the head back, looking up to the fingers. Hold for one minute or more, breathing deeply (figure 2).

- Then bring the head forward and reverse the hand and wrist positions. Repeat in changed

position, holding the head back for the same amount of time.

- To release, bring the head forward. Exhale and release the arms to the sides. Relax in Mountain Pose.

Benefits: This pose brings the energy down through both feet, connecting to the Earth. It strengthens the heart, ankles, legs and back. Raising the arms up recirculates energy through the arms and chest. This pose stretches the chest, shoulders, arms, wrists and throat. It relieves the digestive and abdominal organs from pain. The pineal, pituitary, thyroid, thymus and adrenal glands, pancreas and gonads are stimulated.

Chakras: All the chakras are balanced.

Age level: Suitable for ages 3 and up.

Seated Vine Pose
(Ūrdhva Parivṛtta Hasta Gomukāsana)

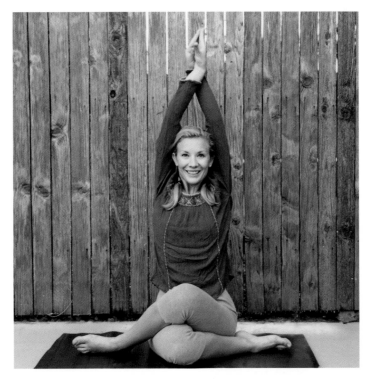

- Start in a seated position with the legs straight out in front, spine straight.

- Cross the left leg over the right, placing the left knee above the right, turning the top of the left foot on the ground, with toes pointing back.

- If the hips are tight, keep the right leg straight out in front with the foot flexed.

- Otherwise, bend the right leg back with the top of the foot resting near the left buttock. At this point the knees are aligned over each other.

- Inhale to raise the arms up overhead, crossing the wrists and turning them in toward each other, palms together. Keep the arms straight with the elbows back behind the ears.

- Hold for one minute or more, breathing deeply. Inhale to straighten the spine, stretching up through the fingers. Exhale to press the sitbones down evenly into the ground, dropping the tailbone, opening the hips. Press the knees down at the same time.

- To release, exhale and relax the arms to the sides of the body. Straighten the right leg out first, then the left. Shake the legs out.

- Repeat to the other side, reversing the leg and hand positions. Hold for the same amount of time.

Benefits: This pose brings the energy down through the buttocks to connect to the Earth. It stretches the ankles, hips, hip flexors, spine, arms, shoulders and wrists. It opens the chest and increases lung capacity, strengthening the back. The reproductive organs are toned. The pineal, pituitary, thyroid, thymus and adrenal glands, pancreas and gonads are stimulated.

Chakras: All the chakras are balanced.

Age level: Not suitable for ages 5 and under. Suitable for ages 6 and up.

Garland Pose
(Mālāsana)

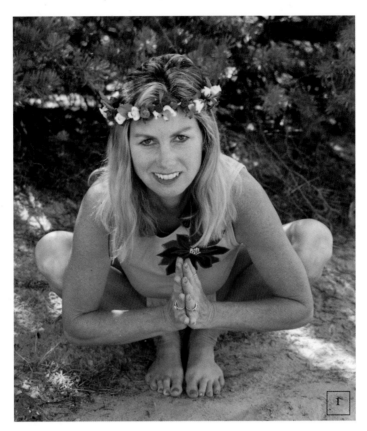

Start in a standing position with the feet together in Mountain Pose (p. 26). Squat down with the feet flat, toes wide. (If the hips are too tight to keep the heels on the ground, place a rolled blanket under the heels for support.)

Level One: Place the palms together and move the chest forward to let the elbows widen the knees. Make sure the feet stay down flat, using the toes and heels for support (figure 1).

Hold this step of the pose for five deep breaths to open the hips. Then exhale to move the torso forward and hold the back of the heels (figure 2).

Level Two: If your knees are wide and your torso is forward with your forehead near the ground, try to go farther to reach around the back of the waist, turning the wrists up, eventually interlocking the fingers (figure 3). (You can hold a strap to bring the hands closer together.)

Hold for one minute or more, breathing deeply. Inhale to stretch the spine out, exhale to move the torso farther forward (eventually bringing the forehead to the ground) and reach farther around the back waist to open the shoulders and upper back.

To release, let the arms relax in front of the body, then inhale to roll the spine up. Sit down and shake the legs out in front. Roll the feet out to stretch the ankles.

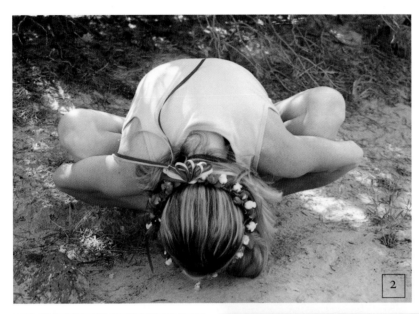

2

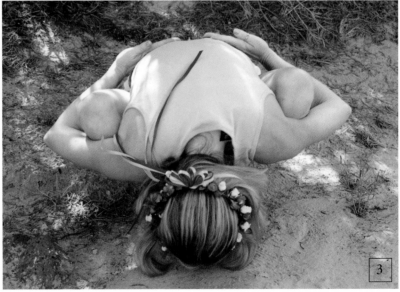

3

Benefits: This pose brings the energy down through the feet and head to connect to the Earth. It strengthens the front of the ankle, leg and heart. It stretches the hips, hip flexors, Achilles tendons, wrists, shoulders, upper and lower back. The blood is moving into the head to relieve headache and clear the mind. The liver, gall bladder, and digestive and abdominal organs are toned. The pineal, pituitary, thyroid, thymus and adrenal glands, pancreas and gonads are stimulated. The kidneys and spleen are relaxed.

Chakras: All the chakras are balanced.

Age level: Level One suitable for ages 3 and up. Other levels suitable for ages 6 and up.

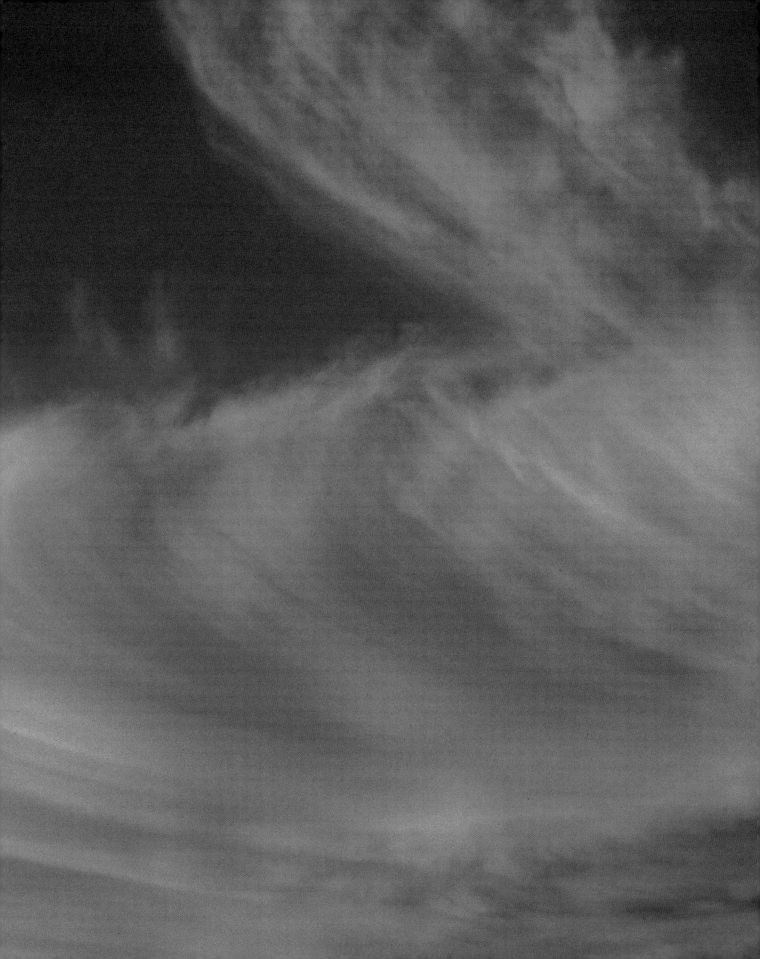

Air

Air poses relate to breathing as well as the constellations that give us a larger sense of the universe. Prana relates to breath or energy and yama to control. Pranayama (a system of breathing exercises) is used to regulate the breath for calming or energizing the nerves, strengthening the lungs and heart, and bringing more oxygen to the brain to clear the mind. Practicing pranayama also balances the chakras, keeping them functioning properly. The poses relating to the sun-sign constellations both bring us closer to our personal power and take the focus off ourselves, placing it instead on the bigger picture, uniting us with the universe.

Primary chakras involved with the Air element
The 4th chakra, Anahata, "unhurt"
The 5th chakra, Visuddha, "sound and ether" (subtle vibrations)
The 6th chakra, Ajna, perception and command center
The 7th chakra, Sahasrara, "thousandfold"

Pranayama

Constellation Poses

"Pranayama is the science of breath. The Yogi's life is not measured by the number of his days but by the number of his breaths."
(B.K.S. Iyengar, Light on Yoga)

Alternate Nostril Breathing
(Nādī Sodhana)

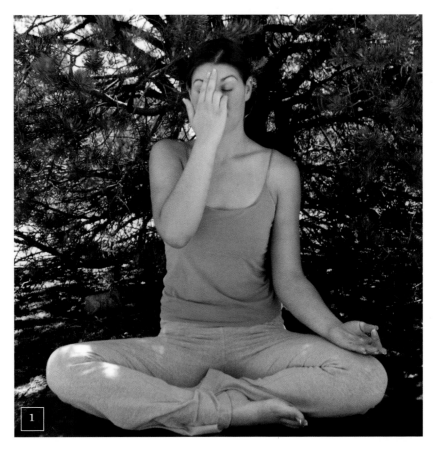

- Start in a seated position in Half or Full Lotus Pose (pp. 22–3) with the spine straight.

- Place the left hand on the left knee with the thumb and index finger touching to create a circle (Jnana Mudra). The thumb represents the universal soul and the index finger represents the individual soul. This circle allows them to connect, creating a balanced being in harmony with the universe.

- Bring the right hand up to the face and let the thumb rest near the right nostril with the middle and index finger stabilized on the forehead at the third eye. The ring finger will touch the left nostril (figure 1).

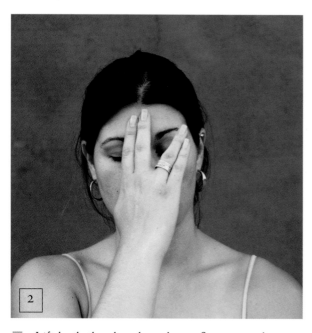

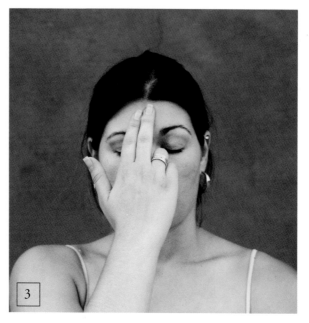

■ Lift both the thumb and ring finger to take a deep breath through both nostrils. Then close the right nostril with the thumb and take a deep breath through the left (figure 2). Close both nostrils and hold the breath, counting to five. Then lift the thumb to exhale through the right nostril (figure 3). Close both nostrils to hold without breath, counting to five. Continue with the inhalation, opening the right nostril, and repeat the pattern.

■ Think of the breath running through the Ida nadi (channel running to the left side of the spine) and down through the Pingala nadi (right channel). Let this energy run in a horseshoe motion from the base of the spine up to the crown and back down to the base. This will help you stay focused on which nostril to breathe through, alternating with each breath. The inhalation is called Puraka. Holding the breath or holding without breath is called Kumbhaka. The exhalation is called Rechaka.

■ Continue running the energy through the nadis, alternating nostrils for 2–5 minutes.

■ To release, relax both hands on the knees in Jnana Mudra (facing page) and take five deep breaths through both nostrils, running the energy through the Sushumna nadi (center channel).

■ Relax the breath and observe the effects of this breathing exercise.

Benefits: This practice of breath control (pranayama) balances the nervous system, stimulates the spine, and calms and clears the mind. This is good for headache or sinus problems.

Chakras: All the chakras are balanced.

Age level: Not suitable for ages 12 and under. Suitable for ages 13 and up.

Cooling Breath
(Sithalī)

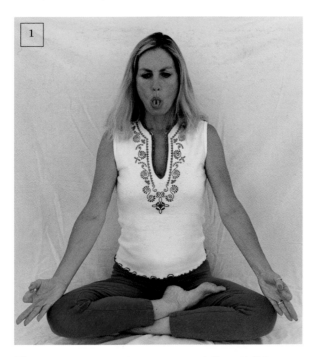

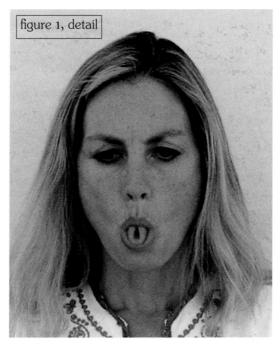

- Start in a seated position in Half or Full Lotus Pose (pp. 22–3) with the spine straight. Place the thumb and index finger together in Jnana Mudra (p. 42) with the back of the hands resting on the knees (figure 1).

- Stick the tongue out and curl it inward from the tip to create a trough. The tongue curling resembles a curled leaf (figure 1, detail). If this isn't possible, make an "O" with the mouth open. Relax the tongue inside the mouth, keeping it inside throughout this exercise.

- Inhale deeply through the mouth with the tongue out, then close the mouth, bring the chin to the chest (Jalandhara Bandha, p. 99) (figure 2) and hold the breath for five counts, tightening the anal sphincter in Mula Bandha (p. 99).

- Lift the head forward to release the chin lock and exhale through the nose (figure 3). This completes one round.

- Repeat 10–25 rounds. Then breathe through the nose to relax, and observe the effects of this breathing exercise.

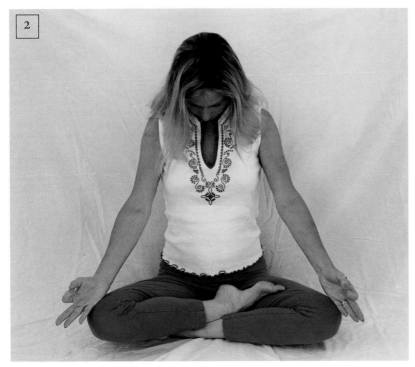

Benefits: This pranayama exercise cools the system like a fan cooling the engine on a car. It relaxes the mind and reduces the heat in the body.

Chakras: All the chakras are balanced, especially the 1st and 5th.

Age level: Not suitable for ages 12 and under. Suitable for ages 13 and up.

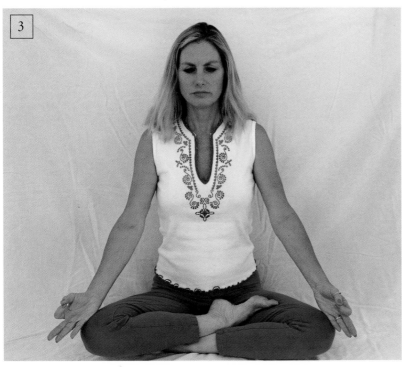

Breath of Fire
(Kapālabhāti)

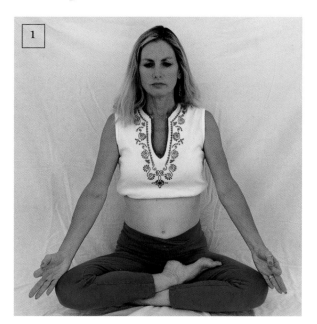

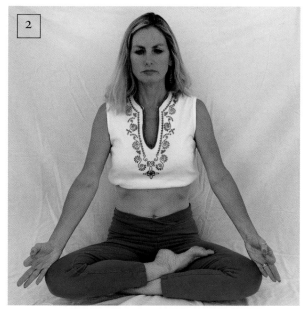

- Start in a seated position in Half or Full Lotus Pose (pp. 22–3) with the spine straight. Place the hands on the knees or abdomen and stay focused on the movement of the belly.

- Breathing through the nose with the mouth closed, take a deep breath to cleanse the lungs (figure 1). Start slowly with inhalations expanding the belly and exhalations contracting the abdominal muscles, pulling them straight back toward the abdominal wall (figure 2).

- Be careful not to move the upper chest or shoulders—the breath stays in the abdomen.

- Build up the pace if you understand the breathing. Count your breaths for 25–50 counts. (A complete breath—inhalation and exhalation—is one count.)

- To release, take 5–10 deep breaths and relax. Observe the effects of this breathing exercise.

Benefits: This pranayama exercise stimulates the internal fire and builds heat in the body. It strengthens the abdominal muscles and stimulates the digestive and reproductive organs. It opens the energy blocks to the brain, clearing the mind and stimulating the nerves. It energizes the body and mind.

Chakras: All the chakras are balanced, especially the 3rd.

Age level: Not suitable for ages 12 and under. Suitable for ages 13 and up.

Deep Breathing
(Ujjayi)

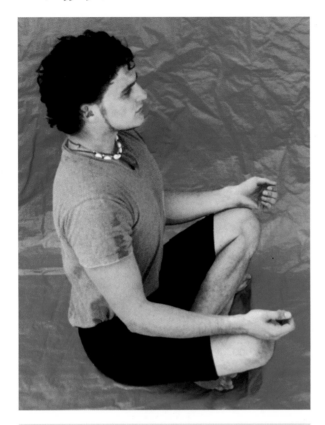

Benefits: *This pranayama breath cleanses and strengthens the lungs, throat and mind.*

▓ Start in a seated position in Half or Full Lotus Pose (pp. 22–3) with the spine straight. Rest the palms on the knees or hold the thumb and index finger in Jnana Mudra (p. 42) with the fingers creating a circle.

▓ Lift the chin slightly with the head forward. Open the mouth wide and take a few deep breaths in and out, listening to the "ha" sound created through the back of the throat. Now close the mouth and practice breathing through the nose, with the breath moving through the back of the throat as if the mouth were still open to create the "ha" sound.

▓ The epiglottis (a lid over the trachea) is closing slightly to make that throaty sound. Use Ujjayi breathing while practicing the asanas or poses. It enables the breath to flow deeper and slower.

▓ Try 10–25 Ujjayi breaths and then relax the breath, focusing on the breaths moving the energy from the base of the spine up the Sushumna (center channel) to the crown on the inhalations. The exhalations move the energy back down the spine to the base.

Chakras: All the chakras are balanced.

Age level: Not suitable for ages 12 and under. Suitable for ages 13 and up.

Aries (Ram), Half Warrior III Prep Pose
(Ardha Vīrabhadrāsana III Prep)

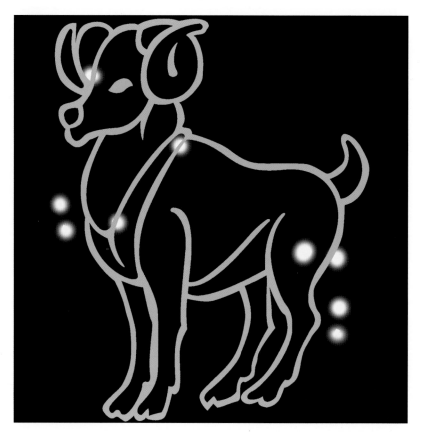

■ Start on the hands and knees with the palms flat under the shoulders, fingers wide and pointing directly forward. The knees are placed under the hips with the spine long.

■ *Level One:* Focus on a spot in front and concentrate. Straighten the left leg out on the ground behind you. Take a deep breath, exhale to lift the left leg up and straight back from the hip, with the toes pointed. Feel yourself grounded through both hands and left shin. The top of the right foot and front of the ankle stay down on the ground, with the big toe pointing straight back. If the back is weak,

stay with this step and breathe deeply. Lengthen the spine and stretch back through the left leg.

■ *Level Two:* If the back is strong in Level One, lift the right arm with the hand straight out from the shoulder, palm facing down.

■ Hold for one minute or more, breathing, deeply. Inhale to lift the chest and straighten the left arm, exhale to stretch back through the left leg, balancing on the right knee and shin, and stretch out through the right arm.

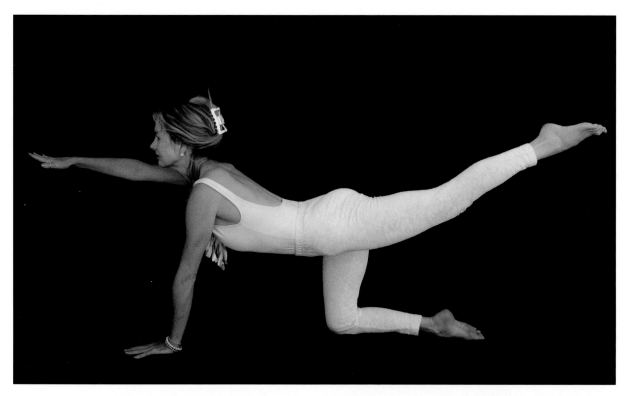

- To release, exhale and lower the right arm down first, and then the left leg. Repeat to the other side and hold for the same amount of time.

- To relax, sit back on the heels with the forehead down, arms to the sides of the body in Child's Pose (pp. 58–9).

Benefits: This balance pose strengthens the shoulders, back, and supported hip and leg. It stretches the chest, outstretched arm and front of the extended leg. It relaxes the belly and strengthens the heart. Holding the balance develops concentration and strengthens the mind. The pineal, pituitary, thyroid, thymus and adrenal glands, pancreas and gonads are stimulated.

Chakras: All the chakras are balanced.

Age level: Level One suitable for ages 3 and up. Level two suitable for ages 6 and up.

Taurus (Bull), Cow's Head Pose
(Gomukāsana)

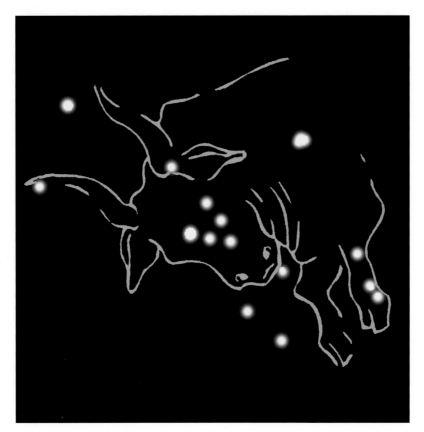

- Start in a seated position with the legs straight out in front, spine straight.

- Cross the left leg over the right, placing the left knee above the right, turning the top of the left foot on the ground, with toes pointing back.

- If the hips are tight, keep the right leg straight out in front with the foot flexed.

- Otherwise, bend the right leg back with the top of the foot resting near the left buttock. At this point the knees are aligned over each other.

- Place both hands behind the back. Hold the right forearm with the left hand and climb up the back with the right hand, fingers pointing up, wrist turned out.

- Inhale to raise the left arm overhead and drop the left hand back to eventually grasp the right. If the

shoulders are too tight and the hands won't reach, hold a strap between the hands (figures 1 and 2).

- Hold for one minute or more, breathing deeply. Inhale to lift up through the left elbow, moving it behind the head. Exhale to pull down through the right arm. Let the breath help you stretch farther, opening the right shoulder and chest.

- To release, let go and rest the arms to the sides. Straighten the left leg out and then the right. Shake the legs out and roll the shoulders.

- Repeat to the other side, reversing the leg and arm positions, and hold for the same amount of time.

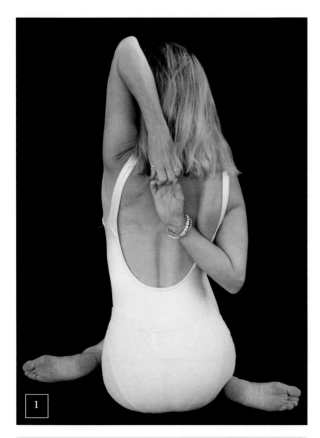

1

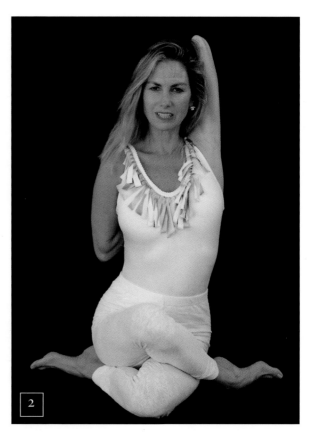

2

Chakras: All the chakras are balanced.

Benefits: This pose stretches the ankles, hips, hip flexors, belly, chest and shoulders. It strengthens the upper back and helps correct stooped shoulders. It opens the lungs and relaxes the digestive organs to relieve discomfort in the belly. The abdominal and reproductive organs are toned. The pineal, pituitary, thyroid, thymus and adrenal glands, pancreas and gonads are stimulated.

Age level: Not suitable for ages 5 and under. Suitable for ages 6 and up.

Gemini (Twins), Partner Squats Variation Pose
(*Utkaṭāsana* Variation)

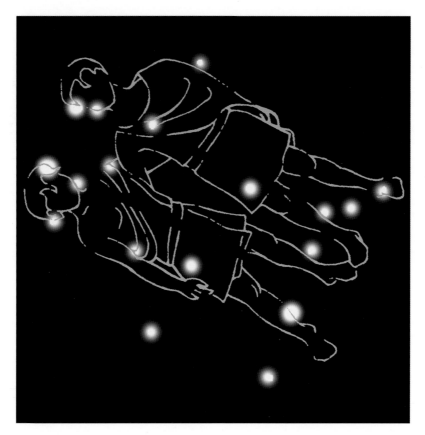

■ Partners begin by standing back to back. Keep the feet hip-width apart, toes wide and forward with the heels a few inches away from each other.

■ Reach back with the arms to hook around your partner's arms with the elbows bent.

■ Together decide when you will begin. Then take a deep breath and exhale, pressing against each other's backs, and slowly squat down as far as you can, keeping the backs straight (figure 1).

■ Hold as long as you can, breathing deeply, then decide together when it is time to come up. Then inhale to push the backs against each other and use the legs to rise slowly to a standing position (figure 2). (This sounds easier than it is!)

■ Release the arms to the sides and take a deep breath to relax.

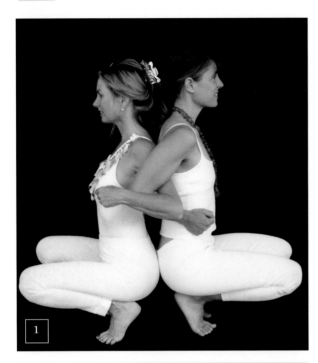

1

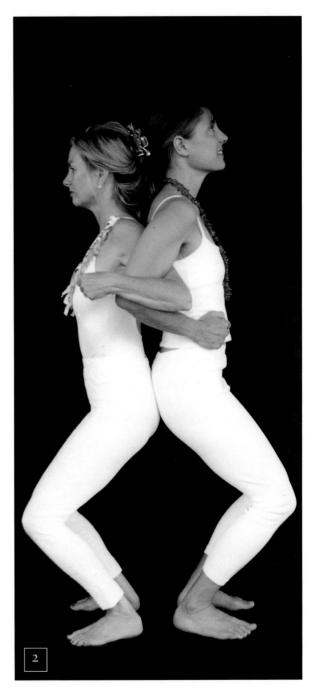

2

Benefits: This pose strengthens the mind, back, heart, hips, legs, ankles and toes. It opens the chest and stretches the shoulders and Achilles tendons. It tones the abdominal and reproductive organs. The mind's concentration on the intense effort necessary to complete this pose enhances motor skills. The pineal, pituitary, thyroid, thymus and adrenal glands, pancreas and gonads are stimulated.

Chakras: All the chakras are balanced.

Age level: Not suitable for ages 5 and under. Suitable for ages 6 and up.

Cancer (Crab), Crab Pose
(*Pūrvottanāsana* Prep)

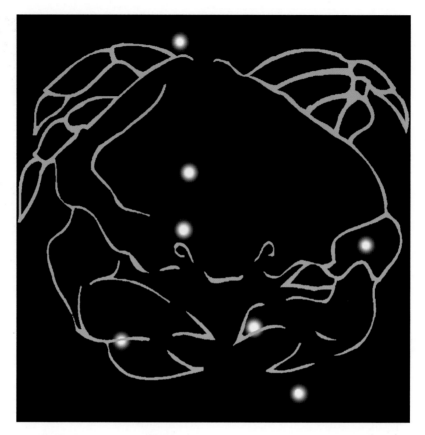

■ Start in a seated position with the legs bent, feet hip-width apart, toes turned in slightly and resting flat on the ground close to the buttocks.

■ *Level One:* Place the hands under the shoulders, palms flat, fingers wide, turned toward the knees. Open the chest and roll the shoulders down and back.

■ Take a deep breath, exhale and lift the pelvis as high as you can. Bring the head back. Lengthen out through the knees with the tailbone tucked, and move the weight back through the feet. The knees are aligned over the heels at a right angle (figure 1).

■ Hold for one minute or more, breathing deeply. Open the chest and lift the pelvis on the inhalations, press out through the knees and down through the feet on the exhalations. The weight needs to be distributed evenly through the hands and feet by lifting the pelvis. Press the thighs in, knees hip-width apart. If there is too much weight on the wrists due to a weak back (not being able to lift the pelvis high enough), then release down slowly from here.

■ *Level Two:* If you are strong in Level One, try a leg lift. Keep the pelvis lifted and straighten the left leg out on the ground. Exhale to lift it up as high as you can in the air and flex the foot. Hold for five deep breaths, making sure the right knee doesn't fall out to the side (figure 2).

- Exhale to release the left leg straight down with the heel to the ground and bend it in.

- Repeat, lifting the other leg, and hold for the same amount of time.

- To release, exhale and slowly sit down. Release the arms, straighten the legs out in front and shake them out. You can lean forward over both straight legs to stretch the back out.

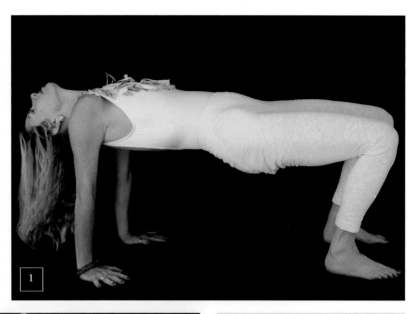

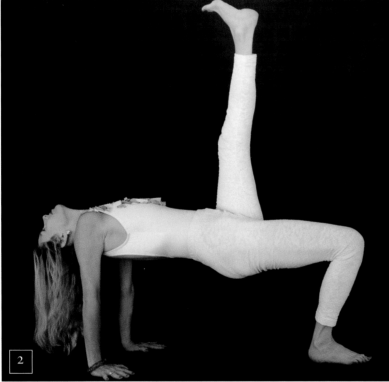

Benefits: This pose strengthens the arms, shoulders, wrists, fingers, back, buttocks, hamstrings, ankles and toes. When the leg is lifted, the back of the leg is stretched and concentration is required to balance, strengthening the mind. It stretches the entire front of the body. This relieves pressure from the digestive organs and reproductive organs. It opens the lungs and heart. The spleen, kidneys and nervous system are stimulated. The pineal, pituitary, thyroid, thymus and adrenal glands, pancreas and gonads are stimulated.

Chakras: All the chakras are balanced.

Age level: Level One suitable for ages 3 and up. Level Two suitable for ages 6 and up.

Leo (Lion), Lion Pose
(Siṃhāsana)

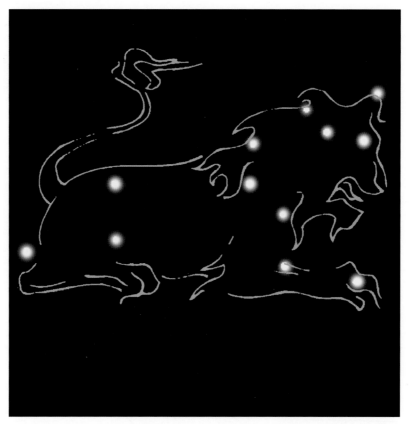

Start in a seated position in Half or Full Lotus Pose (pp. 22–3) with the spine straight. (This pose can be done in either leg position; however, Full Lotus Pose is where you eventually want to be.)

Place the hands in front of the legs on the ground, palms flat, fingers wide and directly forward.

Take a deep breath and exhale to press down through the hands to lift the buttocks off the ground and balance on the knees (figure 1). (If you are in Half Lotus Pose, the bottom leg will fall back.)

Start walking the hands forward and press the pelvis down toward the ground. Lift the sternum, dropping the shoulders away from the ears to open the chest.

Now begin your "Lion's breaths." Take a deep breath, inhaling through the nose and exhaling through the mouth with the tongue out, looking up to the third eye (figure 2). Close your eyes and mouth to repeat your inhalation, then exhale, again looking up with your tongue out. (Be careful not to force the exhalation and hurt your throat. Let it be slow and gentle.)

Repeat 5–10 Lion's breaths. To release, walk the hands back in and ease the buttocks to the ground. Sit with the spine straight and take a deep breath.

Release the leg position slowly and reverse it. Go back through the steps to move forward, walking the hands out and pressing the pelvis down toward the ground.

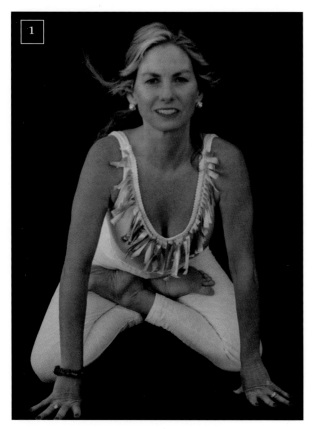

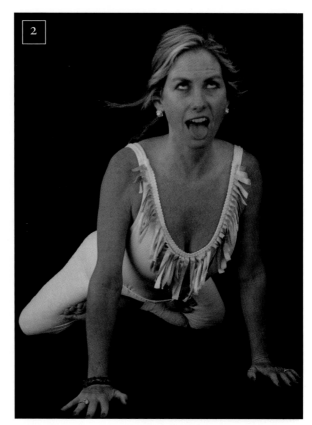

- Repeat the same number of Lion's breaths. Then walk the hands back, placing the buttocks on the ground. Sit with the spine straight and take a deep breath.

- Release the legs and shake them out. Roll the feet in circles to stretch the ankles.

Benefits: This pose stretches the ankles, hips, hip flexors, front of the spine, chest, shoulders, arms, wrists, face and eyes. It strengthens the back and neck. It relaxes the digestive and abdominal organs, while it stimulates the heart, lungs, kidneys and mind. The Lion's breath is excellent for relieving a sore throat or bad breath. The pineal, pituitary, thyroid, thymus and adrenal glands, pancreas and gonads are stimulated.

Chakras: All the chakras are balanced.

Age level: Not suitable for ages 5 and under. Suitable for ages 6 and up.

Virgo (Virgin), Child's Pose
(Bālāsana)

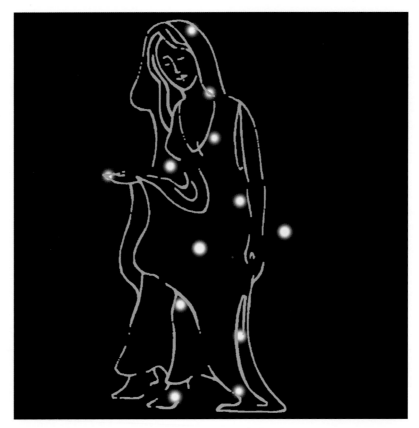

■ Start on the hands and knees. Sit back on the heels and rest the forehead on the ground with the spine lengthened forward, arms resting to the sides of the body.

■ If it is difficult to sit on the heels, fold two blankets and place one under the top of the ankle and one over the back of the ankle. This will lift the buttocks and take some pressure off the knees.

■ This is a relaxation position, but many areas of the body are opening. Try to focus on each area and breathe into it to "let go."

■ Focus on rolling the front of the shoulders down. Open the upper back, moving the shoulderblades away from the spine to open the heart center.

■ Focus on the lower back opening, "letting go" through the sacrum and hips.

■ Feel each vertebra opening and separating through the entire spine. Relax the neck and head.

■ Hold for one minute or more, breathing deeply to focus on opening the back of the lungs.

■ To release, inhale and roll the spine up slowly to sit on the heels. Sit with the legs turned out to each side. Straighten the legs out in front and shake them out.

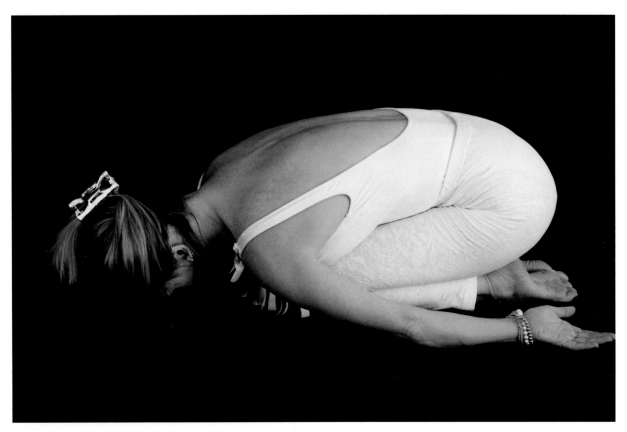

Chakras: All the chakras are balanced.

Age level: Suitable for ages 3 and up.

Benefits: This pose is restorative and very relaxing. It stretches the back, hips and spine. It brings the blood forward to tone the heart, liver, and the digestive, abdominal and reproductive organs. It relieves pressure from the kidneys and spleen. The pineal, pituitary, thyroid, thymus and adrenal glands, pancreas and gonads are stimulated.

Libra (Balance), Shoulder-and-Arm Balance Pose
(Bhujāsana)

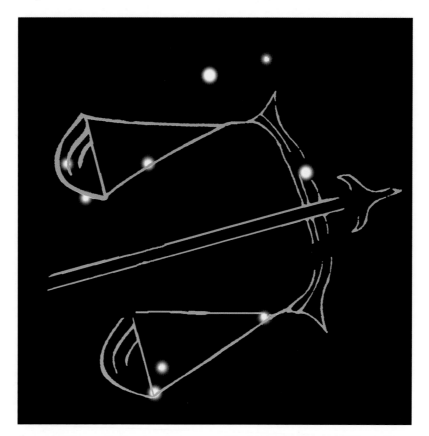

■ Start in a standing position with the feet hip-width apart and squat. Reach the arms down between the legs and place the palms flat on the ground to the outside of each foot. The fingers are wide and pointing directly forward (figure 1).

■ Sit back slightly to release the feet from the ground and try to bring the soles together.

■ The hamstrings rest on the triceps with the knees reaching toward the shoulder. Straighten the arms and try to balance (figure 2).

■ Hold for one minute or more, breathing deeply. Lift the sternum on the inhalation and balance strongly through the hands on the exhalation.

■ To release, bring the feet down to the ground, slide the arms out and sit down to relax. Shake the legs out and take a deep breath.

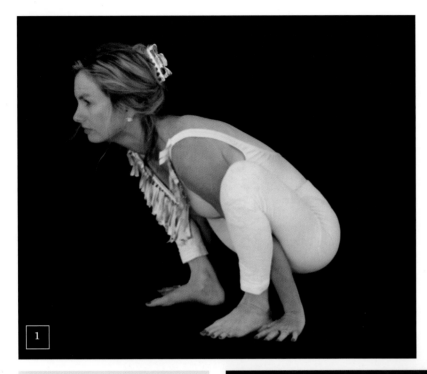

1

Chakras: The 1st, 2nd, 3rd, 4th, 6th and 7th chakras are balanced.

Age level: Not suitable for ages 5 and under. Suitable for ages 6 and up.

Benefits: This balance pose strengthens the wrists, arms, shoulders and back. It stretches the hips and hip flexors. It stimulates the liver, digestive, abdominal and reproductive organs. Balancing on the hands develops concentration to strengthen the mind. The pineal, pituitary, thymus and adrenal glands, pancreas and gonads are stimulated.

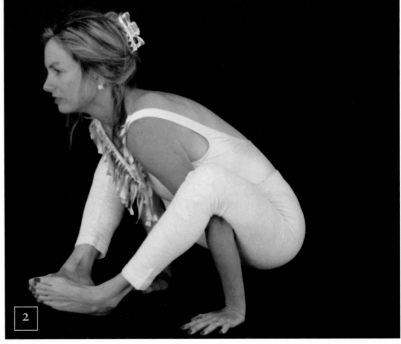

2

Scorpio (Scorpion), Scorpion Prep Pose
(Vṛśchika)

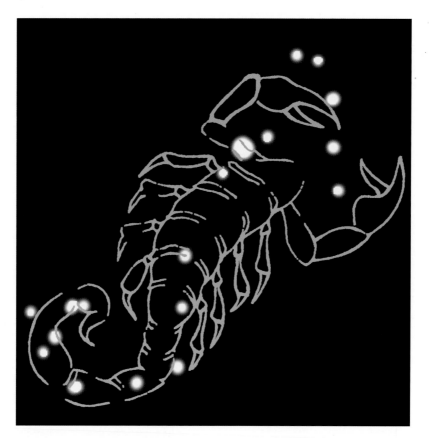

■ Start on the hands and knees with the knees under the hips. Place the forearms on the ground, with the elbows under the shoulders. Run a straight line from the elbow to the index finger and widen the thumbs to create a rectangle between them. Widen the other fingers and press down. Make sure the wrists stay down.

■ Curl the toes under and exhale to lift the knees up from the ground and straighten the legs. Take a few deep breaths, then lift the shoulders and tailbone to the sky on the inhalations. Press the chest back toward the thighs and down toward the heels on the exhalation. Stretch the spine and the back legs, and look toward the feet with the neck in line with the spine.

■ Now, exhale and lift the right leg straight up in the air with the hips even. Rise to the toes of the left foot and exhale to bend the right foot back toward the buttock. Press the right knee up toward the sky to stretch the quadriceps.

■ Hold for one minute or more, breathing deeply. Inhale to lift the shoulders and rise higher in the left foot, then exhale to bend the right foot back and lift the knee higher, pressing down evenly through the forearms and hands.

■ To release, straighten the right leg, then bring the left foot down flat. Take a deep breath and exhale to lower the right leg slowly.

■ Repeat to the other side and hold the same amount of time. To release, sit back on the heels in Child's Pose (pp. 58–9).

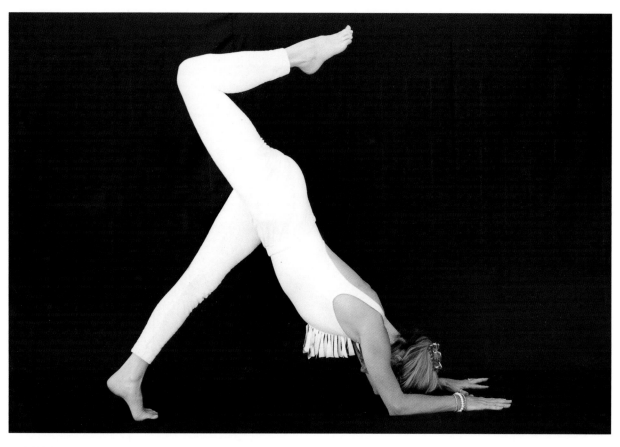

Chakras: All the chakras are balanced.

Age level: Not suitable for ages 5 and under. Suitable for ages 6 and up.

Benefits: This inverted pose reverses the blood flow into the upper body to strengthen the heart and mind. It is good for headache, apathy and sinus problems. It strengthens the arms, wrists, shoulders, and back and front of the standing leg. It stretches the front thigh of the upper leg and back of the standing leg. Releasing the neck forward relieves tension and separates the cervical vertebrae of the neck. The digestive, abdominal and reproductive organs, liver, spleen, kidneys and nervous system are stimulated. The pineal, pituitary, thyroid, thymus and adrenal glands, pancreas and gonads are stimulated.

Sagittarius (Archer), Dancer's Pose
(Nātārājāsana)

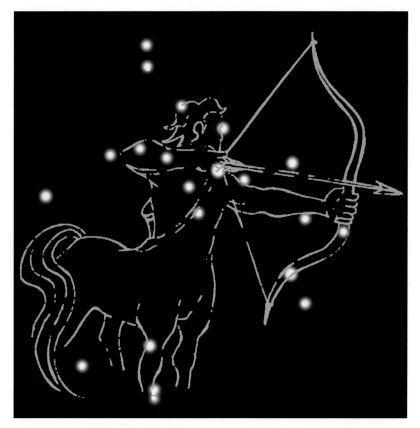

- Stand with the feet together and arms to the sides in Mountain Pose (p. 26). Take a deep breath to get grounded.

- Focus on one spot in front, exhale to bend the right leg straight back and hold the top of the right foot with the right hand. Keep the knees aligned and facing front. Inhale to reach the left arm up with the elbow beside the ear. Keep the left leg tight.

- Take another deep breath and exhale to move the torso forward about 30 degrees. Balance on the left foot, toes wide, and concentrate. Begin lifting the right thigh back, moving the foot away from the buttock.

- Hold for one minute or more, breathing deeply. Each time you exhale, try to lift the right leg higher behind you. The hips stay forward with the right thigh looking down toward the ground. (Don't twist the lower back.)

- To release, exhale and slowly lower the right leg. Stand with the feet together, straighten the spine and release the left arm down. Take a deep breath, realigning in Mountain Pose.

- Repeat to the other side and hold for the same amount of time.

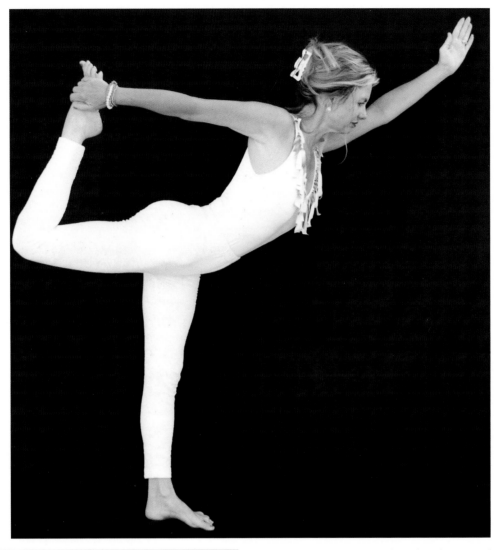

Chakras: The 1st, 2nd, 3rd, 6th and 7th chakras are balanced.

Age level: Not suitable for ages 5 and under. Suitable for ages 6 and up.

Benefits: This balance pose strengthens the standing ankle, leg and hip. It strengthens the back while stimulating the kidneys. It relaxes the digestive organs. It stretches the ankle and quadriceps of the bent leg as well as the chest, arms and shoulders. The pose develops concentration to strengthen the mind and eyes. The pineal, pituitary, thymus and adrenal glands, pancreas and gonads are stimulated.

Capricorn (Goat), Hands-and-Knees Lift Pose
(*Ardha Dhānurāsana* Variation)

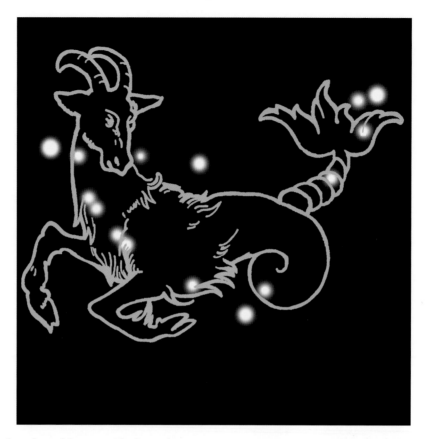

- Start on the hands and knees with the palms flat on the ground, under the shoulders, fingers wide, pointing directly forward. The knees are under the hips with the spine long. Keep the tops of the ankles down with the big toe pointing straight back.

- Take a deep breath and exhale to lift the left leg straight back and up in the air with the hips squared. Breathe deeply and hold this step, focusing on a spot in front.

- Concentrate and exhale to bend the left leg and lift the right hand from the ground to reach back and hold the top of the left foot.

- Hold for one minute or more, breathing deeply. Inhale to lift the sternum and straighten the left arm. Exhale to lift the left leg higher and open the right shoulder.

- To release, exhale and lower the right arm with the hand on the ground. Take another deep breath and exhale to straighten the left leg and slowly lower it, bending the knee in under the hip.

- Take a deep breath and straighten the spine. Repeat to the other side and hold for the same amount of time.

- To relax, sit back on the heels with the arms to the sides, forehead on the ground (Child's Pose, pp. 58–9) and rest.

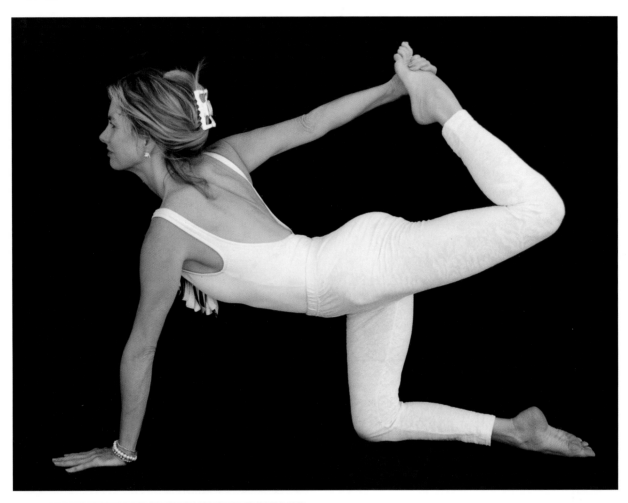

Chakras: All the chakras are balanced.

Age level: Not suitable for ages 5 and under. Suitable for ages 6 and up.

Benefits: This balance pose strengthens the hips, back, buttocks, arms, wrists and shoulders. It stretches the front of the shoulder of the lifted arm, and the front of the leg and ankle of the lifted leg. It requires concentration, strengthening the mind and eyes. The digestive organs are relaxed, while the kidneys and heart are stimulated. The pineal, pituitary, thyroid, thymus and adrenal glands, pancreas and gonads are stimulated.

Aquarius (Water Bearer), Water Wheel Pose
(Ūrdhva Prasārita Pādāsana)

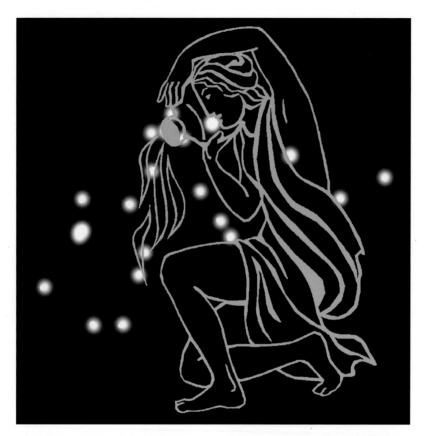

- Start in a supine position on the back. Keep the hips and shoulders even with the spine, aligned on the ground. The arms rest to the sides of the body with the legs together.

- Inhale to bend the knees into the chest (figure 1) and straighten the legs up to the sky, with feet flexed (figure 2).

- Exhale to slowly lower the legs straight down to the ground, keeping the back down (figure 3). (If the lower back hurts, stop midway down and bend the knees to release the legs.)

- This is a flowing pose using deep breathing through the three moves. As the breath deepens, the body slows down with the flow. Stay focused on the body and the breath moving together.

Benefits: This pose strengthens the abdominal muscles, back and legs. It stretches the backs of the legs as they are lowered. It stimulates the digestive and abdominal organs to help digestive problems. The reproductive organs, pancreas, gonads and the adrenal glands are stimulated.

Chakras: The 1st, 2nd and 3rd chakras are balanced.

Age level: Suitable for ages 3 and up.

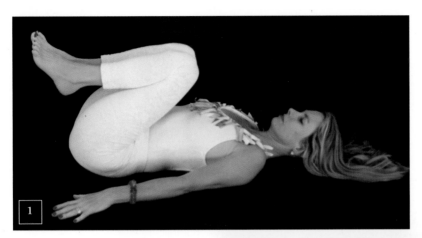

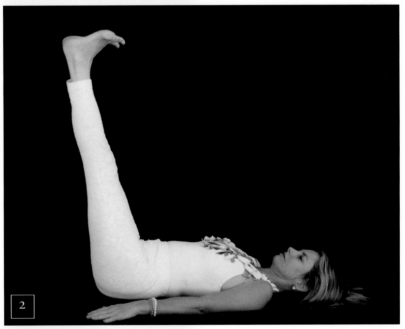

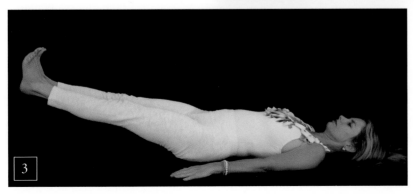

PIsces (Fish), Fish Leg Lift
(Ūttāna Pādāsana)

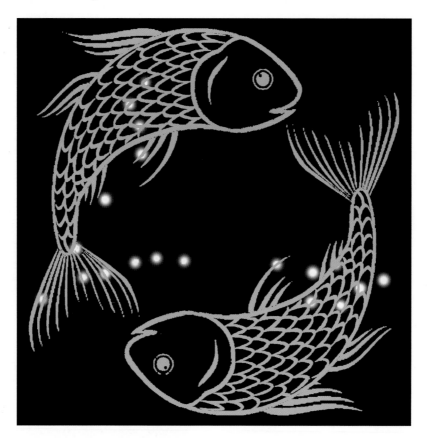

- Start in a supine position on the back. Slide the hands under the buttocks, palms down, arms straight and shoulders pulled down away from the ears.

- Keep the legs together and straight out on the ground with the feet flexed.

- Take a deep breath and push down through the arms and hands to lift the chest (arching the back). Place the crown of the head on the ground (figure 1).

- Release the arms and hands from the ground and place them in prayer position (Anjali Mudra, p. 26) over the abdomen. Make sure the shoulders stay relaxed and down away from the ears.

- Take a deep breath and exhale to lift the legs up from the ground (⅓ to ⅔ of the way to vertical). Point the toes, keeping the legs straight.

- On the next exhalation, straighten the arms out to point the fingers toward the toes (figure 2).

- If it is too difficult at first to raise both legs at the same time, try lifting one leg and holding it for a few breaths. Then release and lift the other leg.

- Hold for one minute or more, breathing deeply. To release, exhale and slowly lower the legs straight down to the ground. Take another deep breath and exhale to bring the arms to the sides of the body on the ground and roll the back down.

- Relax on the back with the knees bent into the chest. Take a few deep breaths.

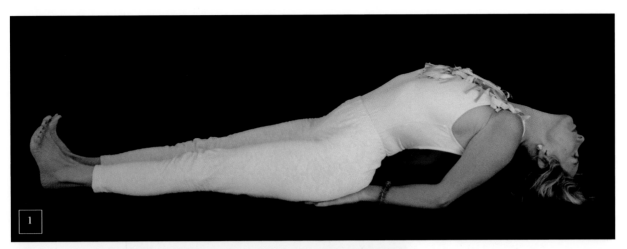

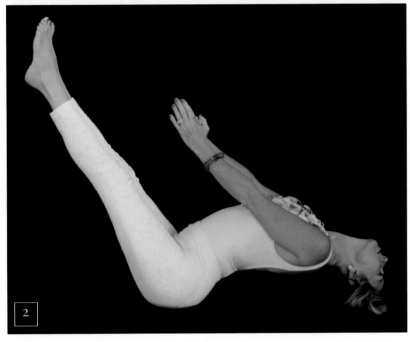

Benefits: This back-bending pose strengthens the back, hips and back of the legs. It stretches the throat, shoulders, arms, belly, front of the spine, front of the legs, ankles and toes. The kidneys are stimulated. The pineal, pituitary, thyroid, thymus and adrenal glands, pancreas and gonads are stimulated.

Chakras: All the chakras are balanced.

Age level: Not suitable for ages 12 and under. Suitable for ages 13 and up.

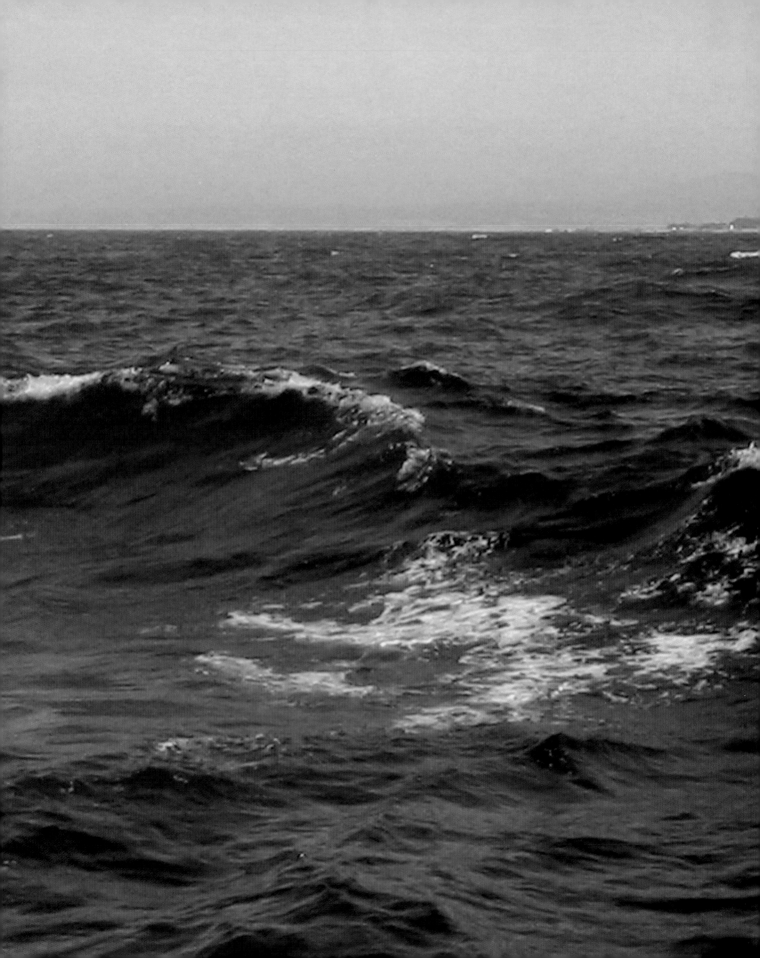

WATER

Water poses reflect the fact that we are mostly water, which enables us to flow and be flexible. Water animals are models for some of these poses; through them we may learn their ability to float through life, free of burdens. Water poses also include waves for experiencing the ebb and flow of life and keeping the spine flexible. These also balance the nervous system.

Primary chakra involved with the Water element
2nd chakra, Svadisthana "one's own place or base"

Water Poses

"Yoga is the method by which the restless mind is calmed and the energy is directed into constructive channels."
(Patanjali, Yoga Sutras)

"Yoga is experienced in nonattachment, that mind which has ceased to identify itself with its vacillating waves of perception."
(Patanjali, Yoga Sutras)

Starfish-on-Wall Pose
(*Vasiṣṭhāsana* Variation)

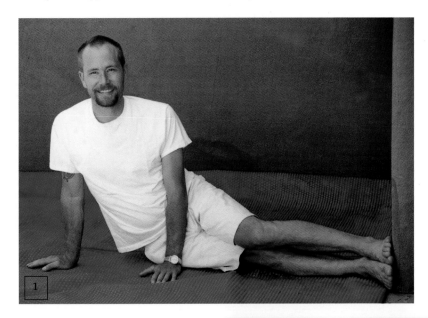

Chakras: All the chakras are balanced.

Age level: Level One suitable for ages 3 and up. Level Two suitable for ages 6 and up.

Benefits: This balance pose strengthens the wrists, arms, shoulders, heart, back, abdominal muscles and legs. It stretches the chest and belly and opens the lungs. The pineal, pituitary, thyroid, thymus and adrenal glands, pancreas and gonads are stimulated.

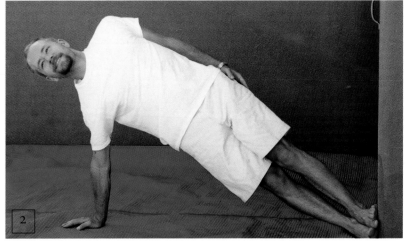

■ Start by sitting with the right side of the body on the ground near a wall with the right palm flat and placed under the right shoulder at a 90-degree angle, fingers wide.

■ Place the feet flat against a wall with the outer edge of the right foot on the ground, left foot resting on top of the right. Keep the legs straight (figure 1).

■ *Level One:* The left hand rests on the ground in front of the hips. Take a deep breath and exhale to lift the right hip, pressing down through the right and left hands, along with the feet. Keep the legs tight with the tailbone tucked. Your body should be a straight line running from the crown of the head through the feet. Bring the left arm to the side of the body. The chest and pelvis stay forward (figure 2).

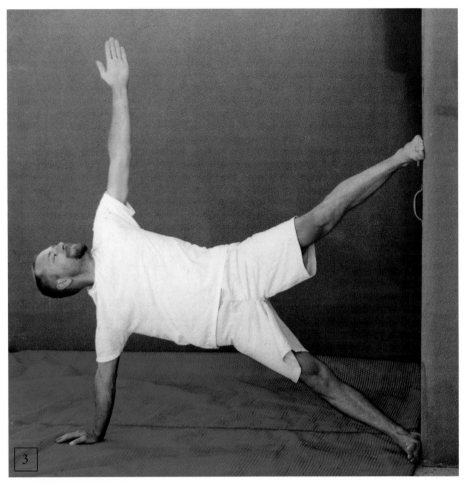

3

- If this step is difficult to hold strongly, stay with it for a few breaths, distributing the weight through the feet so it isn't all on the wrist. Release from here and try again, holding longer.

- *Level Two:* If you are strong in Level One, exhale and raise the left foot up the wall. Keep the left foot directly above the right, pressing the pelvis forward with the tailbone tucked.

- Inhale to raise the left arm with the hand directly up from the shoulder, and look up (figure 3).

- Hold for one minute or more, breathing deeply. Inhale to reach up through the left hand, opening the chest. Take some weight off the right wrist by lifting the right hip and exhaling to press through the legs and feet.

- To release, bring the left leg down to meet the right, then release the left hand to the ground in front of the hips. Bring the body down slowly and take a deep breath.

- Repeat to the other side and hold for the same amount of time.

Seal Pose
(*Mayūrāsana* Prep)

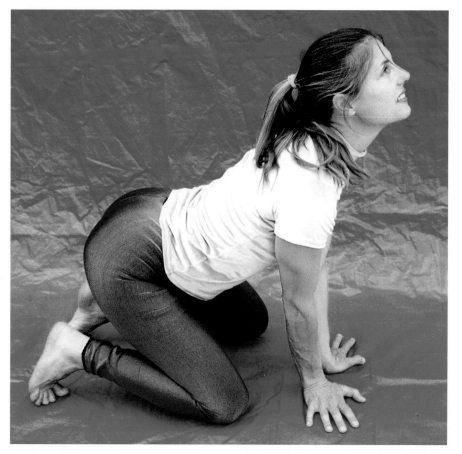

- Start in a seated position on the heels with the toes curled under.

- Place the palms flat, shoulder-width apart, on the ground under the shoulders, fingers wide and turned out to the sides.

- Lift the buttocks off the heels slightly and stretch the throat, lifting the chin. Look up to the third eye.

- Hold for one minute or more, breathing deeply. Inhale to lift the sternum, and exhale to pull the shoulders down away from the ears. Keep the arms straight and press down through the hands.

- To release, sit back on the heels with the spine straight, tops of the feet down. Turn the legs to one side and straighten them out.

Benefits: This pose stretches the toes, wrists, chest, throat and eyes. It opens the lungs. It strengthens the back while it stimulates the kidneys. The pineal, pituitary, thyroid, thymus and adrenal glands, pancreas and gonads are stimulated.

Chakras: All the chakras are balanced.

Age level: Suitable for ages 3 and up.

Seal Race with Ball (group pose)

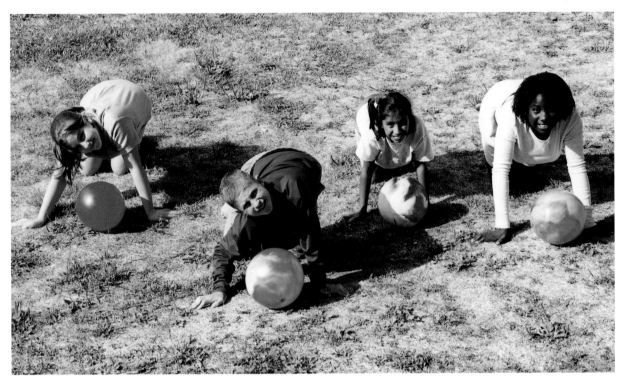

This race can be done with two or more people.

- Start on the hands and knees, lined up side by side in a straight line, with a ball in front of each person.

- Curl the toes under and keep the hands turned out to the sides in Seal Pose (facing page).

- Have someone stand near a finish line and say "Start" to begin the race. Start pushing the ball straight ahead with the nose, scooting forward with the body, keeping the hands out to the sides, and staying close to the ball.

- Push the ball short distances to the finish line, using the neck, arms, back and legs. Feel the heart accelerating.

- Rest once you finish!

Benefits: This race strengthens the entire body and stimulates the heart.

Chakras: All the chakras are balanced.

Age level: Suitable for ages 3 and up.

Dolphin Pose
(Sirṣāsana Prep)

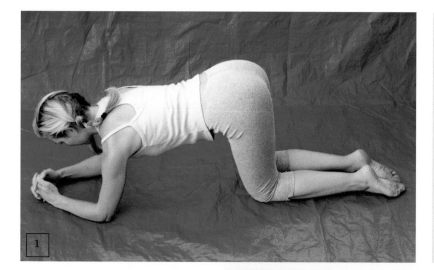

Benefits: This inverted pose strengthens the wrists, shoulders, arms, back and abdominal muscles. It stretches the back of the legs and Achilles tendons. The digestive organs, heart and brain receive a fresh supply of blood. The pineal, pituitary, thyroid, thymus and adrenal glands, pancreas and gonads are stimulated.

Chakras: All the chakras are balanced.

Age level: Level One suitable for ages 3 and up. Level Two suitable for ages 6 and up.

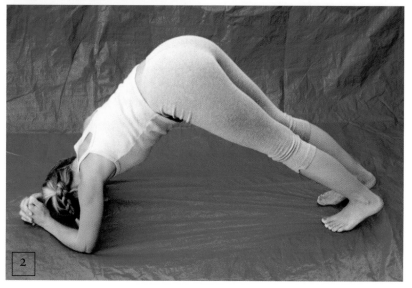

■ Start on the hands and knees with the elbows under the shoulders, fingers interlocked and palms open (figure 1).

■ Place the crown of the head on the ground, holding the back of the head with the open palms, fingers cradling the head. The weight bears down from the outside of the hand to the elbow, through the entire forearm evenly. The wrist bones point toward the sky.

■ *Level One:* Curl the toes under. Take a deep breath and exhale to lift the knees up from the ground and straighten the legs.

■ Exhale and lift the head off the ground, looking back toward the legs (figure 2).

■ Hold for one minute or more, breathing deeply. Inhale to lift the shoulders and tailbone toward the sky, and exhale to press the heels toward the ground.

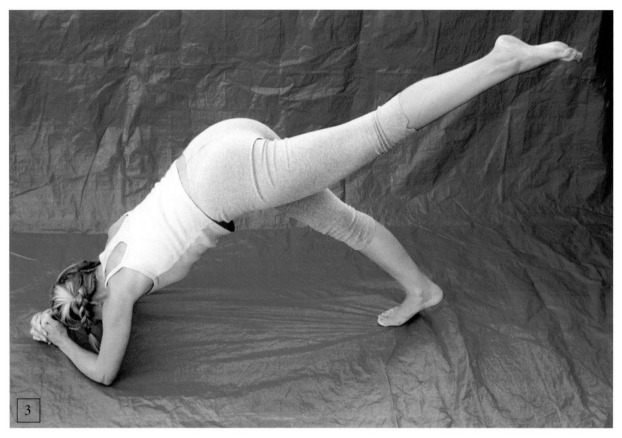

3

- If you do not feel strong in this step, keep practicing with both feet on the ground, head up, to build strength in the upper back and shoulders.

- *Level Two:* If you feel strong in Level One, keep the head off the ground and exhale to lift the left leg straight up in the air with the hips even (figure 3).

- Hold for five or more deep breaths and exhale to release the leg down slowly.

- Take another deep breath and exhale to lift the right leg, holding for the same amount of time. Exhale to release the leg.

- To release the pose, bend the knees, sit on the heels with the forehead down (Child's Pose, pp. 58–9) and rest.

Whale Pose
(*Dhānurāsana* Prep)

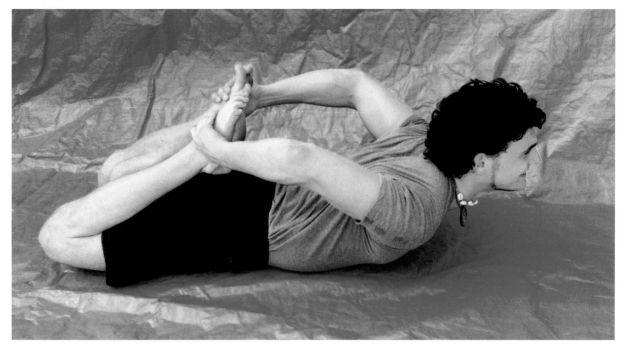

■ Start by lying down on the stomach with the chin down and legs hip-width apart. Place the arms to the sides of the body on the ground.

■ Bend the feet in toward the buttocks. Inhale to lift the chest up, then reach back to hold the tops of the feet.

■ Keep the thighs down, pressing the pelvis down and tucking the tailbone.

■ Hold for one minute or more, breathing deeply. Inhale to lift the chest higher and exhale to bring the feet in toward the buttocks, keeping the thighs and pelvis down.

■ To release, exhale and lower the chest and arms first, then the legs.

■ Relax, lying on the stomach with the head turned to one side.

Benefits: This pose strengthens the back, buttocks and hamstrings. It stretches the chest, shoulders, quadriceps, front of the ankles and toes. The foot position helps build an arch to aid flat feet. The liver, kidneys, and abdominal and digestive organs are toned. The thyroid, thymus and adrenal glands, pancreas and gonads are stimulated.

Chakras: The 1st, 2nd, 3rd, 4th and 5th chakras are balanced.

Age level: Suitable for ages 3 and up.

Resting Whale Pose
(Pārṣva Dhānurāsana)

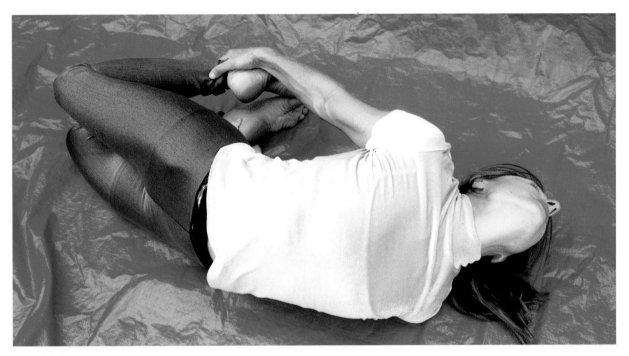

- Start lying on the stomach and move into Whale Pose (facing page).

- Take a deep breath and exhale to roll to the left side by pulling the left shoulder and right thigh back.

- Lift the head off the ground to create a large curve, with the head moving back toward the feet.

- Try to open the chest enough to rest on the front side of the left shoulder. Draw the thighs back, moving the heels away from the buttocks, straightening the arms.

- Hold for one minute or more, breathing deeply. Inhale to open the chest and exhale to bend back.

- Come back to Whale Pose and repeat to other side.

- To release, exhale and lower the chest and arms, then the legs.

- Roll over on the back with the knees into the chest, rocking from side to side to massage the spine.

Benefits: This pose gives the same benefits as Whale Pose. The added benefit is more stretch through the front of the spine, thighs and hip flexors. This pose also stimulates the heart, thymus and thyroid more. The spleen and liver receive more blood when you are rolling to the sides. The pineal, pituitary and adrenal glands, and the pancreas and gonads are stimulated.

Chakras: All the chakras are balanced.

Age level: Not suitable for ages 5 and under. Suitable for ages 6 and up.

Penguin Pose
(Ūtkaṭāsana Variation)

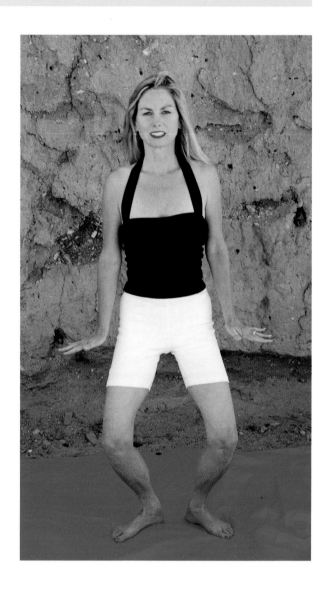

- Start in a standing position with the feet hip-width apart, toes turned to the outside. The arms rest to the sides of the body with the fingers turned out, palms parallel to the ground.

- Push down through the hands to move the shoulders away from the ears.

- Take a deep breath, exhale and bend the knees. Tuck the tailbone as if sitting and press the pelvis forward.

- Hold for one minute or more, breathing deeply. Release the tuck of the tailbone and inhale to open the chest. Exhale to "sit down" a little more, tucking the tailbone to press the pelvis forward.

- To release, inhale and straighten up. Exhale and stand in Mountain Pose (p. 26). Take a deep breath.

Benefits: This pose strengthens the buttocks, back, hips, legs and ankles. It stretches the chest, wrists and hip flexors. The pineal, pituitary, thyroid, thymus and adrenal glands, digestive organs, pancreas and gonads are stimulated.

Chakras: All the chakras are balanced.

Age level: Suitable for ages 3 and up.

Penguin Race (group pose)

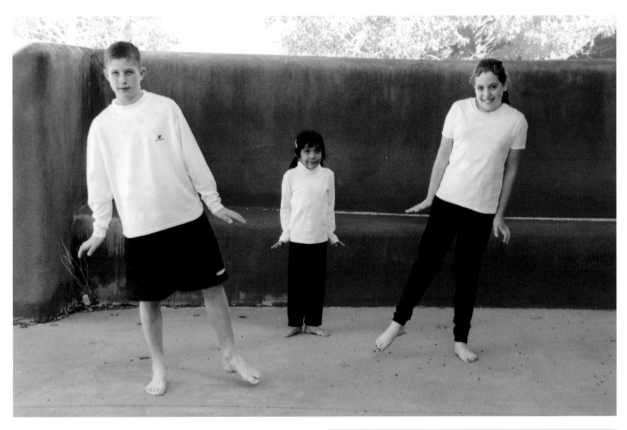

This race can be done with two or more people.

▪ Line up in a straight line, side by side, in a standing position. Tuck the tailbone down as in Penguin Pose (facing page), and keep the legs straight.

▪ To begin the race, have someone stand at a finish line and say "Start." Walk with the legs tight and palms pressing down to keep the chest open and back strong. Move from side to side with the feet turned out like a penguin.

▪ Try walking backward to the "Start" line too! You can also have fun with friends walking in circles without a race.

Benefits: This race stimulates the brain and develops motor skills. It strengthens the back, buttocks, hips, legs and ankles. It stretches the chest and wrists and increases flexibility in the hip joints. The pineal, pituitary, thyroid, thymus and adrenal glands, pancreas and gonads are stimulated. The whole body feels alive and strong!

Chakras: All the chakras are balanced.

Age level: Suitable for ages 3 and up.

Crab Walks Race (group pose)
(*Pūrvottanāsana* Prep)

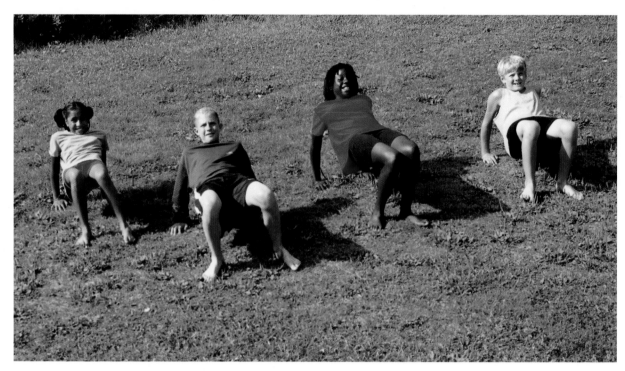

This race can be done as a moving pose for one person or a race with two or more people. It is designed for the young at heart!

■ Line up side by side in a straight line in a seated position with the knees bent, feet hip-width apart, close to the buttocks.

■ Place the hands under the shoulders, palms flat, fingers wide and pointing toward the knees.

■ Take a deep breath and exhale to lift the buttocks off the ground, pressing the pelvis up as high as you can, tucking the tailbone. The knees will be aligned over the heels at a right angle, arms straight.

■ Hold this pose (Crab Pose, pp. 54–5) for a few breaths with the pelvis up.

■ To begin the race, have someone stand at the finish line and say "Start."

■ Begin walking forward, moving the hands and feet as fast as you can and looking forward.

■ Once you get to the finish line, go backward to the starting line then sit down to rest. (You can also walk to the right or left sides, or in circles!)

Benefits: This race strengthens the entire body, stimulates the heart and builds motor skills.

Chakras: All the chakras are balanced.

Age level: Suitable for ages 3 and up.

Snail Pose
(Pīndāsana Prep)

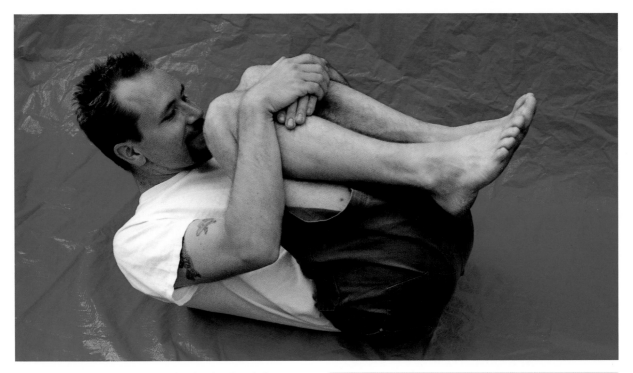

- Start by lying down on the back. Bend the knees into the chest. Wrap the arms around the legs just below the knees.

- Take a deep breath and exhale to lift the head to the knees. (Lift head from the sternum, being careful not to strain the neck.)

- Hold for one minute or more, breathing deeply.

- To release, exhale and roll the back and head down slowly, then let go of the legs. Relax.

Benefits: This pose is used to stretch the back after back-bending or inverted poses. It is very calming to the nerves and a great stretch for the spine. It tones the digestive and abdominal organs and is good for constipation or digestive problems. The thyroid, thymus and adrenal glands, pancreas and gonads are stimulated.

Chakras: The 1st, 2nd, 3rd, 4th and 5th chakras are balanced.

Age level: Suitable for ages 3 and up.

Fish Pose
(Mātsyāsana)

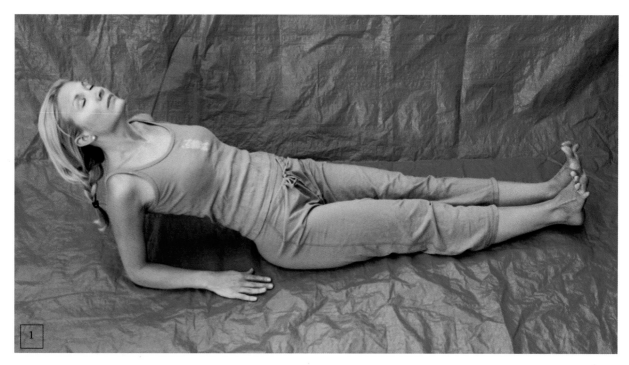

- Start by lying down on the back with the legs straight out in front, feet flexed.

- Place the hands against the buttocks on the ground with the thumbs wide, and stretch back to bring the elbows and forearms to the ground. Keep the legs tight and the feet flexed.

Benefits: This pose strengthens the back and the front of the legs. It stretches the throat, chest, belly and back of the legs. The digestive organs are relaxed while the kidneys are stimulated. It opens the lungs and heart. The pineal, pituitary, thyroid, thymus and adrenal glands, pancreas and gonads are stimulated.

- *Level One:* Inhale to lift the chest up and exhale to bend the back with the shoulders open (figure 1).

- *Level Two:* Place the crown of the head on the ground. If the back is not strong enough to create the bend to get the crown down, stay up higher and breathe into the chest and then release the pose by inhaling to lift yourself up. If your neck hurts, keep the chin to the chest and continue bending back.

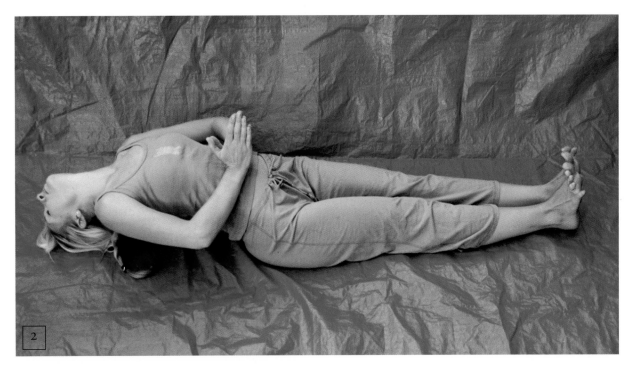

2

- If you are able to hold the pose with the crown on the ground, place the palms in prayer position (Anjali Mudra, p. 26) over the abdomen. (This is your fin.) Make sure the shoulders drop down away from the ears (figure 2).

- Hold for one minute or more, breathing deeply. Inhale to open the chest, then exhale to relax the shoulders and push through the heels.

- To release, lower the arms to the sides of the body and exhale while rolling the back down slowly. Take a deep breath.

- Bring the knees into the chest and rock from side to side to massage the spine. You can also hold Snail Pose (p. 85) for a few breaths to reverse the stretch on the spine.

Chakras: All the chakras are balanced.

Age level: Level One suitable for ages 3 and up. Level Two suitable for ages 6 and up.

Seahorse Pose
(Jaṭhara Parivṛtti Variation)

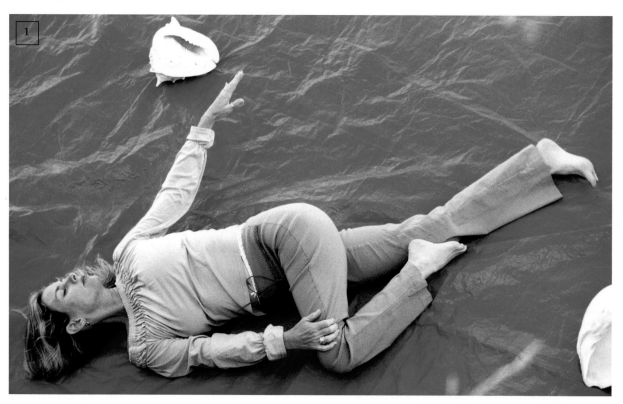

- Start by lying down on the back with the legs together, arms to the sides of the body.

- Place the left foot on top of the right thigh near the knee. Hold the outside of the left knee with the right hand.

- Take a deep breath and exhale to twist the spine and move the hips to the right side, bringing the knee down toward the ground.

- Keep both shoulderblades down while twisting. Tighten the right buttock. Look over the left shoulder (figure 1).

- Exhale and bend the right foot back toward the left buttock, trying to hold the right foot with the left hand (figure 2). (You can use a strap around the foot to hold the foot if you can't reach it with your hand.)

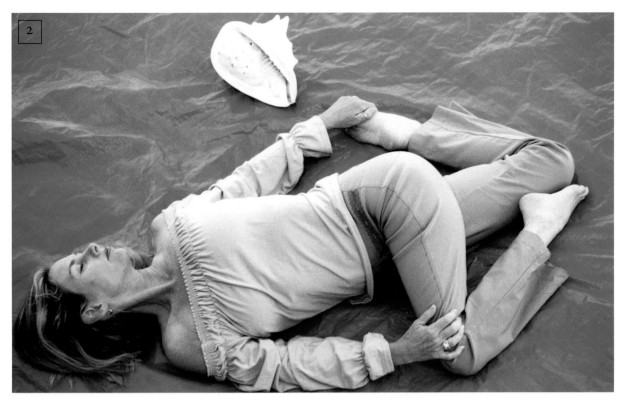

■ Hold for one minute or more, breathing deeply. Inhale to open the chest and exhale to bring the shoulderblades down, twisting farther and trying to move the right thigh back for more stretch through the quadriceps.

■ To release, straighten the right leg and untwist. Move the left leg back to the starting position and relax.

■ Repeat to the other side and hold for the same amount of time.

Benefits: This pose is good for digestive problems or constipation. It strengthens the back and buttock on the bottom leg. It stretches the chest, shoulders, top hip, hip flexors and ankles. The digestive organs, kidneys, spleen, liver and spine are stimulated. The thyroid, thymus and adrenal glands, pancreas and gonads are stimulated.

Chakras: The 1st, 2nd, 3rd, 4th and 5th chakras are balanced.

Age level: Not suitable for ages 5 and under. Suitable for ages 6 and up.

Partner Octopus Pose
(*Hālāsana* Variation)

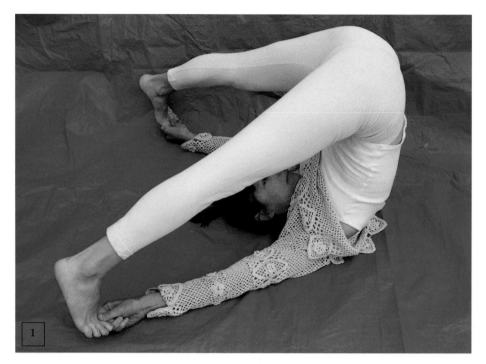

This pose can be practiced alone or with a partner. If practicing alone, follow the same steps. Instead of pressing the soles of your feet against your partner's and holding hands, hold onto your own toes with the legs wide (figure 1).

■ Start by lying down on the back with your head facing your partner's head. Position yourself so that when you extend your arms straight back overhead on the ground, you are able to grasp your partner's hands.

■ Bring the arms to the sides of the body, keeping feet together and legs tight.

■ Let your partner know when you are ready for the next step and do it at the same time. Take a deep breath and exhale to lift both legs straight up toward the sky at a 90-degree angle.

■ Take another deep breath and exhale to swing the hips up with the legs overhead and toes to the ground. Try to keep the spine straight.

■ Take a few deep breaths. Inhale to lift up through the tailbone and exhale to push out through the heels.

■ Interlock the fingers behind the back on the ground and pull the shoulders down away from the ears to lengthen the neck. (If the neck hurts, place a folded blanket under the shoulders so the head rests on the ground lower than the shoulders.)

■ Once aligned in this position, reach the arms straight out overhead on the ground and hold your partner's hands.

■ Now widen and straighten the legs to press the soles of the feet against each other's (figure 2).

■ Hold for one minute or more, breathing deeply and helping your partner to keep the toes pointed toward the ground. (If this isn't possible, each person can hold onto his own back and keep the feet out across from the

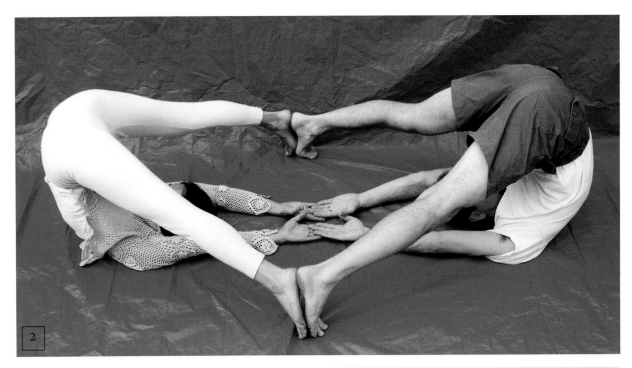

2

hips, legs straight, trying to press the soles of the feet against each other's.)

■ To release, move the arms behind the back on the ground. Lift the legs together overhead, keeping them straight and close to the front of the body. Exhale to roll the spine down slowly, separating each vertebra, rolling one at a time, until the buttocks are on the ground with the legs straight up at a right angle, feet flexed.

■ Align the spine onto the ground, exhale to press through the heels and lower the legs slowly. Bend the knees in to the chest and rock from side to side to massage the spine. Release the legs to the ground and relax.

Benefits: This pose stretches the spine, arms, and back of the legs. It strengthens the front of the legs, abdominal muscles, upper back and neck. The blood is reversed into the upper body to stimulate the heart, liver and brain. The digestive organs and spine are also stimulated from being upside-down. The pineal, pituitary, thyroid, thymus and adrenal glands, pancreas and gonads are stimulated.

Chakras: All the chakras are balanced.

Age level: Not suitable for ages 5 and under. Suitable for ages 6 and up.

Waves I: Rolling Situps Pose
(Rolling *Kūrmāsana*)

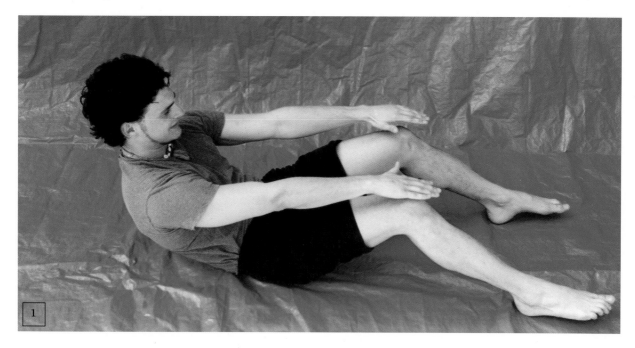

1

- Start in a seated position with the knees bent, feet flat on the ground about 2 feet away from the buttocks and hip-width apart.

- Keep the spine straight with the arms extended in front of the chest. Tuck the chin to the chest.

Benefits: This pose separates each vertebra to plump the discs and stimulate the nerves, opening energy blocks to the brain by clearing the central channel (Sushumna). It strengthens the abdominal muscles and builds arches to help flat feet. The digestive organs and kidneys are toned. The pineal, pituitary, thyroid, thymus and adrenal glands, pancreas and gonads are stimulated.

- Take a deep breath and exhale to roll the back of the spine down slowly (figure 1), stopping at the shoulderblades, looking forward. Take two deep breaths (figure 2).

- Inhale to slowly lift the torso up to straighten the spine. Exhale and stretch forward through the legs (figure 3).

- Repeat your waves, rolling the spine down and up 5–10 times, breathing deeply.

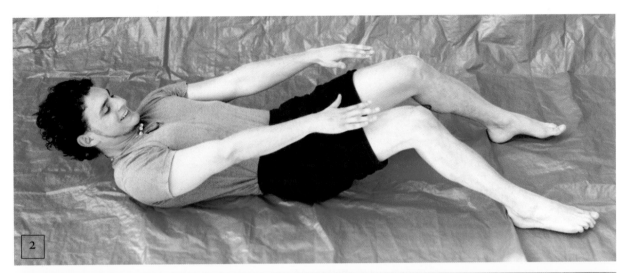

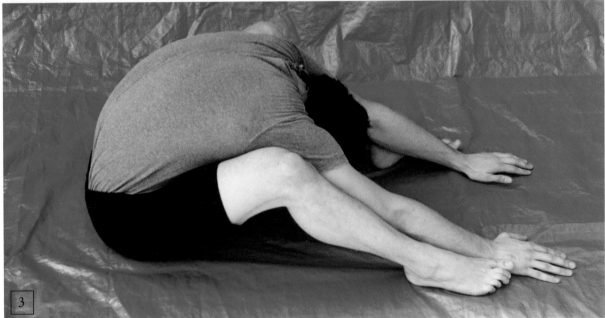

Chakras: All the chakras are balanced.

Age level: Not suitable for ages 5 and under. Suitable for ages 6 and up.

Waves II: Hands-and-Knees Pose
(Rolling *Bhujāngāsana*)

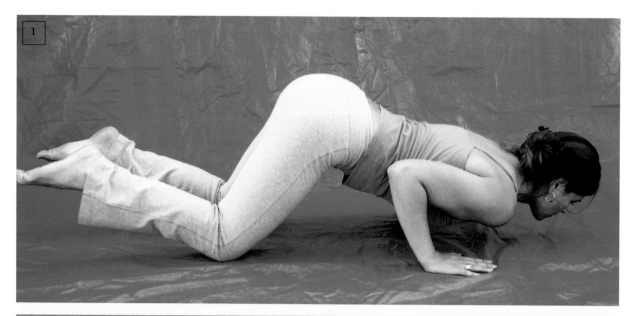

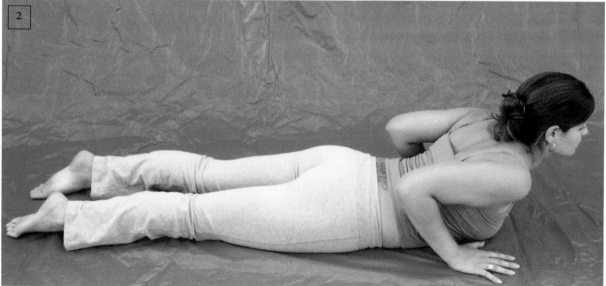

■ Start on the hands and knees, with the hands placed under the shoulders, fingers wide and pointing directly forward. The knees are under the hips with the spine long.

■ Take a deep breath, exhale and bend the elbows into the sides of the body, lowering the head and chest down toward the ground (figure 1). Let the chin, chest, belly and legs move down in sequence as you lower the entire front of the body to the ground (figure 2).

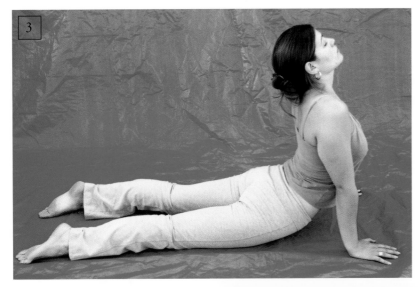

Chakras: All the chakras are balanced.

Age level: Not suitable for ages 5 and under. Suitable for ages 6 and up.

Benefits: This pose strengthens the wrists, arms, shoulders, back, buttocks and back of the leg. It stretches the spine, chest, front of the leg and ankle. The kidneys, spleen, liver, reproductive organs, digestive organs, and nervous system are stimulated. The pineal, pituitary, thyroid, thymus and adrenal glands, pancreas and gonads are stimulated.

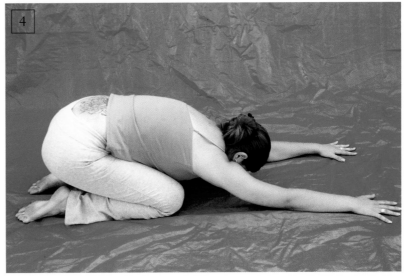

■ Inhale to slowly lift the head and chest up to a Cobra position with the arms straight, shoulders dropping away from the ears and chest open. Look up to the third eye (figure 3).

■ Exhale and lift the buttocks to stretch the back, sitting on the heels, arms extended overhead on the ground (figure 4).

■ Breathe deeply to repeat these flowing waves 5–10 times, opening the front of the spine.

Savasana
(Relaxation)

Savasana (*Śavāsana*) is a position for relaxation. It is important to practice this at the end of each yoga session. Start by lying on the back and begin Abdominal Breathing (below).

With the front of the body open, rest the arms alongside the waist on the floor, palms turned up. Visually draw a line down the center of the body from the head through the spine. Then visualize two parallel lines running along the centerline, and allow the shoulders, hips and heels to rest along the parallel lines. Relax the arms and let the feet fall open.

As the body continues to relax with each abdominal breath, feel yourself sinking into the Earth. Don't hold on to any part of the body or mind. . . . *Let go.*

Abdominal Breathing

Focus on the softness of the breath and rhythmic movement of the abdomen rising on the inhalation and collapsing on the exhalation. The diaphragm moves downward from the ribcage to press the abdomen toward the sky when inhaling. When exhaling, the diaphragm moves back up under the ribs to release the expansion of the abdomen.

A Sample Visualization

Here is a sample visualization. You can use this one or one of your choosing. Let your heart open, release any tightness in the chest and any judgment in the heart and mind that you have been holding onto. Visualize Mother Earth's massive, gentle hands cupping your body to support you physically and emotionally, soothing your soul. Surrender yourself fully to Her and observe how light you feel. Now feel the front of your body opening to Father Sky above you. Surrender yourself fully to Him, feeling light and open.

Visualize an eagle feather hovering high above you in the sky. Experience the lightness and freedom of this feather, as it slowly floats down, eventually landing on your heart.

Focus on the breath flowing in and out. Let go of any worldly concern and let the mind relax deeply into the emptiness.

When you are ready, take a deep breath and feel energy circulating through the body. Visualize energy moving up the spine (through the *Sushumna*) from the 1st chakra to the 7th chakra at the crown. Exhale and send a white light back down the spine, stimulating and balancing all the chakras. This white light represents pure, positive energy.

Visualize white light spreading vital energy through all the channels *(nadis)* within the body. The nadis have been cleared from your asana practice. Feel all energy blocks released from the internal body.

Now visualize this white light seeping through every pore of the skin. Let it form a protective shell or cocoon around the external body, preventing negative energy from entering your psyche or body. Negative energy manifests as disease—mental or physical. Continue lying still, completely relaxed, all cares released, for as much time as you have.

To end, take a deep breath and feel the body realigning and strengthening as you slowly begin to move and stretch. Draw the knees into the chest slowly. Roll to the left side (the moon, or emotional, side) in fetal position, resting. Then slowly roll to the right side (the sun, or linear, side), again resting. Help yourself up to a seated position with the spine straight and take a deep breath. Reconnect with the Earth, blending with nature, balanced through the center.

This relaxation exercise should take five to ten minutes, but it can last longer if you have the time.

"The soul that moves in the world of the senses and yet keeps the senses in harmony finds rest in quietness."
(Bhagavad Gita)

THE SCIENCE OF YOGA

Yoga is the oldest system of personal development in the world. It unites the body, mind and spirit. The term *yoga* means "union." Ancient yogis had a keen understanding of the nature of mankind and what it takes to live in harmony with oneself and one's environment. They thought of the body as a vehicle, the mind as the driver and the soul as the true human identity, combining three forces—action, emotion and intelligence—to pull the body-vehicle. It is important for these three forces to be in balance for full development. The yogis developed a system to maintain this balance, using the poses (asanas) for physical health as well as breathing (Pranayama) and meditation to create peace of mind.

Yoga practice has become popular throughout the world. One of the most popular paths is hatha yoga. More and more people are being taught hatha yoga as a means of rendering the body and mind a fit vehicle to enhance the spirit.

Hatha yoga is the practice of combining asana and breath. Hatha literally means "sun" (*ha*) and "moon" (*tha*)—the polarization of the sun and moon blending to create a balanced being. In practicing yoga poses, the body and mind join to build strength, flexibility, balance and concentration and to align with nature. The classical poses were named after animals, which the sages studied to learn their secrets of staying strong and healthy. Out of these studies sprang a series of poses that imitate the behavior and stance of animals and are designed to create similar agility, poise and determination. Poses imitating inanimate objects or natural features were also developed.

Poses (asanas) tone the body internally and keep the muscular structure strong. As one holds a pose, the blood bathes a particular area of the body to rejuvenate glands and cells and calm the nerves. Some yoga poses are designed for energizing and some are for calming and focusing. Because of these effects, yoga is looked upon as a healing art, not just an exercise program.

The union of body and mind experienced while practicing hatha yoga creates mental as well as physical flexibility. The mental training extends beyond the physical effects, enabling us to cultivate an open and positive attitude and become more rational, compassionate human beings.

Over the years, many styles of hatha yoga have developed. Some of the more classical styles provide a physically softer approach to asana work. These include Kripalu, Integral, Sivananda and Viniyoga yoga. Among the more rigorous styles are Iyengar, Astanga and Bikram yoga.

Whatever the style, it is important to remember that the science of yoga is more than just practicing poses—although that is a good place to start. Besides hatha yoga, classical yoga offers four other paths.

Karma yoga is the yoga of action, which teaches us to act unselfishly and with honor. If we watch our actions and their results carefully, we can develop the insight and awareness that increase our sensitivity to everyone and everything around us.

Bhakti yoga is the path of devotion, enabling us to practice the power of love through prayer, chanting and singing. Bhakti yoga draws on our capacity for love and faith and helps us stay connected to something beyond ourselves for hope and enlightenment.

Jnana yoga is the yoga of the knowledge or wisdom that brings us into unity with God. This higher power can be celebrated in any form we choose to relate to. Yoga is not a religion and therefore does not dictate any theological view. Jnana yoga allows us to delve into our true nature or identity for self-realization. Students are encouraged to integrate hatha and karma yoga—to become strong in body and mind and learn selflessness— before going on to the quest for self-realization.

Finally, *raja yoga* is defined as the "royal road" or "king" of yoga practice. It blends mental and physical energy into all-encompassing spiritual energy that leads us to a profound sense of wholeness and the experience of arriving in our spiritual "home"— the place of infinite peace within ourselves.

In the *Yoga Sutras* Patanjali teaches the "eight limbs" of raja yoga, progressive disciplines that purify the mind and body spiritually. They are: *yamas, niyamas, asanas, pranayama, pratyahara, dharana, dhyana* and *samadhi*.

Yamas consist of five moral injunctions that are essential to spiritual development: non-harming (*ahimsa*), truthfulness (*satya*), non-greediness (*aparigaha*), moderation (*brahmacharya*) and non-stealing (*asteya*).

Niyamas are the observances that enable us to move deeper into the purification process: purity (*saucha*), contentment (*samtosa*), austerity (*tapas*), self-study (*svadhyaya*) and constant living in awareness of divine presence (*vara prandhara*).

Asanas are the poses incorporating the body and breath to make us physically strong and flexible.

Pranayama is the practice of regulating the breath to cleanse the body and mind.

Pratyahara is the practice of drawing the senses inward to still the mind in preparation for *dharana* and *dhyana*.

Dharana is the practice of concentration to strengthen the mind.

Dhyana is meditation for mental clarity.

Samadhi is a state of superconsciousness that relieves the body and mind from physical or mental restraints.

Whatever path of yoga we practice, some of its most important lessons for personal growth are opening the mind, developing mental flexibility, letting go of the ego and mastering selflessness.

The Gunas

According to the yogic system, three qualities termed *gunas* exist within any form of energy. Awareness of these qualities is important in our personal development through yoga practice. These are the qualities:

Sattva (purity or goodness) leads to clarity, mental serenity and the divine. It is associated with kindness to others, parenting and meditation. The elements air and water are considered sattvic.

Rajas refers to activity, passion, and the process of change and willfulness. It is associated with pregnancy, moving, indulging in the arts and utilizing creative energy. Rajas stands between the qualities of *sattva* and *tamas*. Earth is considered rajasic.

Tamas tends toward the demonic and refers to darkness, inertia and ignorance. Tamasic behavior includes being overweight, overindulging in any way, and being angry or violent. Fire is considered tamasic.

Every person possesses all three gunas, although one quality will be most apparent or predominant.

When energy takes a form in nature, one of the three qualities predominates, but the other two are also present. As a vegetable grows in a garden, part of it is ready to harvest (sattvic), while some of it is still in the process of growing (rajasic) and some of it is overripe or even rotten (tamasic). If someone commits a crime, the action would be considered rajasic, but the motive could be tamasic, sattvic or rajasic, depending on the details of the situation.

Nadis, Bhandas & Pranayama

Nadis

A nadi is a channel that energy (*prana*) flows through. There are many thousands of nadis running throughout the internal body, dispersing energy from the chakras. The three main nadis run vertically through the torso. The center nadi is the

Sushumna, which runs through the spinal column. The right and left nadis correspond to the sympathetic ganglia of the spinal cord. The right nadi, the *Pingala,* is related to the sun side of the body, representing the linear thinking process. The left nadi, the *Ida,* is related to the moon side of the body and the emotions. *Kundalini* is a dormant or static cosmic energy represented by a coiled snake. It is located at the base of the spine in the 1st chakra and is activated by pranayama or asana practice. When the dormant kundalini is awakened, it moves up the spine through the *Sushumna* to stimulate the seven chakras.

Bandhas

A bandha is an internal lock used to direct energy to specific locations in the body for healing purposes. There are three main bandhas:

Mula Bandha is the Root Lock (p. 99), obtained by tightening the anal sphincter and perineum, which directs energy up to the navel to stimulate the 1st and 2nd chakras along with the related glands and organs .

Uddiyana Bandha is the Navel Lock (p. 11), obtained by pulling the abdominal muscles back toward the lower spine, which circulates energy to the 3rd chakra and the related organs and glands.

Jalandahara Bandha is the throat lock, obtained by bringing the chin to the chest to direct energy into the 3rd, 4th and 5th chakras and all the organs and glands related to them.

Pranayama

Prana relates to "energy" and *yama* is "control." Pranayama (pp. 41–47) is used to regulate the breath for calming or energizing the nerves, strengthening the lungs and bringing more oxygen to the brain to clear the mind. Practicing pranayama also balances the chakras, keeping them functioning properly.

"Yoga is not for him who gorges too much, nor for him who starves himself. It is not for him who sleeps too much, nor for him who stays awake. By moderation in eating and in resting, by regulation in working and by concordance in sleeping and waking, yoga destroys all pain and sorrow."
(Bhagavad Gita)

"Work alone is your privilege, never the fruits thereof. Never let the fruits of action be your motive; and never cease to work. Work in the name of the Lord, abandoning selfish desires. Be not affected by success or failure. This equipoise is called yoga."
(Bhagavad Gita)

MEDITATION & CONCENTRATION PRACTICES

There are many forms of concentration (*dharana*) and meditation (*dhyana*) practice. One can practice either alone or in a group setting. Meditating alone is a peaceful and rewarding experience. Meditating in a group is a very different experience, because it feeds off the array of energies arising within the group. The group energy may be experienced as a resonance, somewhat like the vibration that resonates throughout one's being following the ringing of a gong or bell.

It is best to meditate in a quiet setting. Some people enjoy lighting incense or burning sage or candles to create a peaceful atmosphere. This also clears negative energy from the space you are using for your meditation.

Choose a form of meditation that works for you at any particular time, spending 10 minutes or longer at first, building up to as much as one hour eventually. Here are four practices to try:

Walking Meditation
Physically active, yet relaxed concentration (*dharana*).

The walking meditations are fun alone or in a group. Feeling the elements of earth, air and possibly water (if you are near a river or lake) while walking outdoors gives the body and psyche a fresh splash of therapy, soaking up the elements. The lungs open easily and deeply when the body is active and circulation is stimulated. The body's activity circulates vital energy through the energy channels (nadis). This is a full body-and-mind experience to enjoy.

Waking Meditation
Eyes open with the mind relaxed (*dharana*).

Waking meditation allows you to calm the mind but keep your awareness of the external setting you are in. This meditation is a beautiful visual experience if you are outdoors watching the clouds, earth, campfire or water—getting in touch with any of the four elements in nature. It is a good place to start if you have trouble relaxing the mind. Meditation is not as scary or unfamiliar to the novice when the eyes are open.

Either sit with the legs crossed comfortably and spine straight or lie down on the back or stomach in Savasana. Keep the eyes open and try to relax the body and mind, staying focused on each breath you take. Observe the difference in quantity and quality of each breath. Do the meditation for 10 minutes or longer to enjoy the peace and renew the body and mind.

Floating Meditation
Enjoying weightlessness and relaxed mind (*dhyana*).

Allowing the body to be supported and suspended in water (preferably warm) can provide a feeling of total abandonment and surrender. If you do not own a floatation tank, a bathtub or warm swimming pool works very well.

Seated or Reclining Meditation

Eyes closed with mind relaxed (*dhyana*).

The seated or reclining meditation with the eyes closed provides a deep internalized experience (pratayahara). If it is difficult for you to relax the mind, stay focused on each breath you take. Eventually you can let go of any focus and let the mind go where it will. Surrendering fully to this meditation will awaken your deeper consciousness, and you may experience a sense of a higher power.

Calming the mind, body and spirit to attain the benefits from meditation is a learned practice, like flexibility. As you continue meditating, you may experience the 6th and 7th chakras radiating energy. Keep practicing to reap the full benefits, staying present with all that you are experiencing and feeling. The education you will receive is unlike any other experience in life.

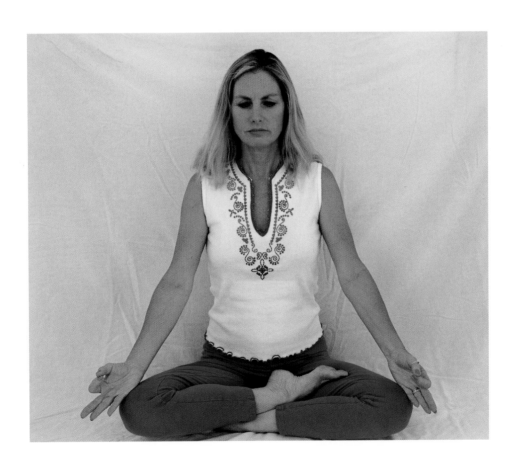

Chakra Energy Centers

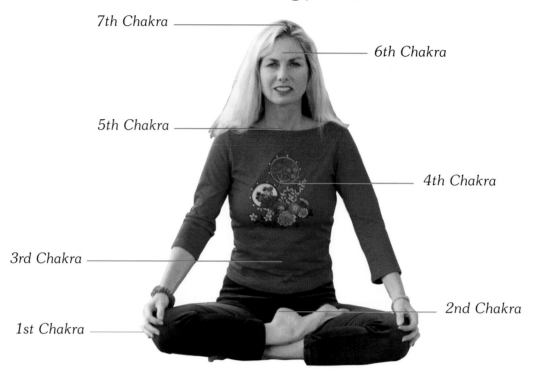

7th Chakra ——————

6th Chakra ——————

5th Chakra ——————

4th Chakra ——————

3rd Chakra ——————

2nd Chakra ——————

1st Chakra ——————

Chakra	Gland	Gland Functions	Parts of Body Affected	Areas & Energy Enhanced When Chakra Energized
1st Base of spine	Adrenals	Secretes hormones that regulate energy output and manage physical and mental stress	Spinal column, central nervous system, legs	Earth. Energy grounding to the Earth, physical body support, independence, stable energy
2nd Sacrum	Gonads	Reproductive glands (testes and ovaries)	Pelvis, large intestine, appendix, bladder, kidneys	Water. Creativity, desire pleasure, sexual energy
3rd Solar plexus	Pancreas	Produces insulin and enzymes to aid in digestion	Digestive organs, liver, gall bladder, small intestine	Fire. Emotional centeredness, self-esteem, personal honor, the emotional seat
4th Heart level	Thymus	Produces infection-fighting white blood cells	Heart, circulatory system, lungs	Air. Love, compassion, trust, loving energy
5th Throat	Thyroid	Makes hormones that help regulate body metabolism and growth	Bronchial tubes, vocal cords	Air. Communication skills, personal expression, emotional energy
6th Forehead	Pituitary	Regulates the activity of the endocrine system and houses the optic nerve	Lower brain	Air + Fire. Knowledge and truth, seeing and thinking from the linear (right side) of the body (as related to the nadis, pp. 98–9)
7th Crown of head	Pineal	Produces melatonin, which regulates sleep, mood, puberty and ovarian cycles	Upper brain	Air + Earth. Faith and inspiration, seeing and thinking from the emotional (left side) of the body (as related to the nadis, pp. 98–9)

The Chakra System

The ancient yogis discovered that the energy (electricity) that flows through our bodies is regulated by centers they termed *chakras*. *Chakra* literally means "wheel." A chakra is an energy center with a circular shape that spins constantly like a wheel, with spokes radiating many colors. However, for simplicity, the main chakras are usually represented by conventional colors that can easily be visualized.

In addition to the line of seven chakras running through the spinal column, there are thousands more chakras sprinkled throughout the internal body. We can think of the chakras as nature's wonders, like stars in the night sky. The thousands of chakras in the body are similar to the billions of stars clustered to make up a galaxy.

The seven main chakras allow different types of energy to enter and spread throughout the body and maintain the balance of emotional and physical strength. When a chakra is in balance, it spins clockwise.

The Chakras & the Four Elements

1st chakra, Muladhara ("root"): Earth

This chakra is positioned at the base of the spine and is a circle of red light. It is the grounding energy—becoming strong, stable and connected to the Earth. Its function is to ground us to our survival needs, take good basic care of the body and purge wastes. The spine, legs, feet and central nervous system are affected by this chakra.

Symptoms of imbalance:
> Deficient: tripping or falling, excessive weight gain as an attempt to ground oneself
> Overactive: greed, hoarding of possessions or money

2nd chakra, Svadisthana ("one's own place or base"): Water

This chakra is positioned at the sacrum and is a circle of orange light. It is the energy governing flow within the body—circulation of blood and lymph, urination, menstruation, orgasm and tears. Its function is to help us open up to pleasure, allowing us to learn to "go with the flow" with moves or changes. The hips, sacrum, lower back, genitals, large intestine, bladder and kidneys are affected by this chakra.

Symptoms of imbalance:
> Deficient: fear of pleasure, being out of touch with feelings, resisting change
> Overactive: running life based on sexual needs or desires

3rd chakra, Manipura ("lustrous gem"): Fire

This chakra is positioned at the solar plexus and is a circle of yellow light. It is the energy of internal fire, heat and light—vitality to move from the strength of the core. Its function is to help us get in touch with self-esteem, our warrior energy, and assume responsibility in life. The digestive organs are affected by this chakra.

Symptoms of imbalance:
> Deficient: inability to set limits, fear, lack of drive to get things done
> Overactive: obsessive need to feel power and gain status or recognition

4th chakra, Anahata ("unhurt"): Air

This chakra is positioned at the heart center and is a circle of green light. It is the energy of love and compassion, wholeness or being complete—opening to air for inspiration and vitality in life. Its function is to help us to get in touch with feelings involving love or acceptance. The heart and lungs are affected by this chakra.

Symptoms of imbalance:
  Deficient: shyness, loneliness, inability to forgive, lack of empathy, shallow breathing, asthma, lung diseases
  Overactive: tendency to use abusive language, brag, argue

5th chakra, Visuddha ("pure or purification"): Air

This chakra is positioned at the throat and is a circle of blue light. It is the energy of the voice and how it is used to communicate freely and openly from the heart. The thyroid and parathyroid glands are affected by this chakra.

Symptoms of imbalance:
  Deficient: fear of speaking, stiff neck, shoulder tension, teeth grinding, jaw disorders, underactive thyroid
  Overactive: yelling, excessive talking, inability to listen, hearing problems, stuttering and overactive thyroid

6th chakra, Ajna ("perception center"): Air/Fire

This chakra is positioned at the third eye and is a circle of indigo (combination of blue and purple). It is the energy of increased perception, insight and imagination. Its function is to help us to get a better understanding of ourselves and how to relate to the world around us in a positive way. The optic nerve and pituitary gland are affected by this chakra.

Symptoms of imbalance:
  Deficient: poor memory, eye problems
  Overactive: headaches, nightmares, problems concentrating

7th chakra, Sahasrara ("thousand-fold"): Air/Earth

This chakra is positioned at the crown of the head and is a circle of violet or white light. It is the opening to the highest state of enlightenment and spiritual development. Its function is to help us to connect to a higher power, looking beyond ourselves to the "bigger picture." The pineal gland is affected by this chakra.

Symptoms of imbalance:
  Deficient: difficulty thinking for yourself, spiritually void
  Overactive: analytical, feeling superior in intellect to others

The Relationship of the Chakras to the Organs & Glands

Ancient yogis discovered that the practice of asanas (poses) could benefit organs and glands by compressing, squeezing and relaxing them through bending, twisting and stretching. The chakras relate to different organs and glands within the body.

1st Chakra

Related organs:

The central nervous system (brain and spinal column) acts as the center for maintaining life. The peripheral nervous system provides communication pathways connecting the central nervous system with the various parts of the body.

Related glands:

Adrenals secrete hormones that regulate energy output and manage physical and mental stress.

2nd Chakra

Related organs:

The large intestine absorbs approximately ¼ of the fluid from the contents from the small intestine. It also absorbs sodium and discharges potassium before passing waste into the rectum. The rectum holds the final processed food before releasing it from the body.

Kidneys, located behind the stomach near the waist, eliminate wastes, regulate the content of water and other substances in the blood, balance electrolytes, and maintain proper salinity balance and alkaline/acid ratio.

The appendix, resembling a fat worm, is the tail end of the juncture of the valve that prevents the contents of the large intestine from flowing back into the small intestine.

Related glands:

The gonads (testes and ovaries) provide hormones during and after puberty to stimulate sexual maturity and regulate the process of reproduction.

The placenta produces hormones necessary for maintenance and growth of the fetus.

3rd Chakra

Related organs:

The stomach begins the process of protein digestion and churns food into paste, storing it for approximately 4 hours before passing it on to the small intestine. The small intestine completes all digestion with the help of the liver and pancreas. It takes approximately 7–9 hours to provide absorption of digested nutrients into the bloodstream.

The gall bladder is a small organ attached to the liver. It stores about ½ of the bile released into the small intestine. The liver produces bile for digestion, extracts toxins and synthesizes nutrients that have been absorbed in the blood.

Related glands:

The pancreas produces strong enzymes that digest protein, fat and carbohydrates, and it produces insulin to regulate blood-sugar level.

The spleen breaks down old red blood cells, removes bacteria and produces lymphocytes (cells essential for immunity).

4th Chakra

Related organs:

The heart is a muscle that contracts and relaxes rhythmically to pump blood through the body

The lungs exchange carbon dioxide for oxygenated blood. The right lung has three lobes and the left lung has two.

Related gland:

The thymus is essential for immunity, producing white cells (T-cells) to attack bacteria, viruses and other foreign substances.

5th Chakra

Related organs:

The pharynx is the tubular part of the throat that connects the nasal and oral cavities. The larynx, which branches off from the pharynx, is the air passageway communicating with the trachea and is the seat of the voice.

The trachea is the tube leading from the larynx into the bronchi, bringing air through and filtering out particles of dust and foreign matter. The bronchi are the branches of tubing that enter the lungs.

Related glands:

The thyroid releases hormones with many functions, including regulating metabolism and growth.

The parathyroid maintains the proper balance of calcium.

6th Chakra

Related organ:

The cerebellum (lower brain) maintains the body's balance and coordinates motor movement.

Related gland:

The pituitary is the primary regulator of the activity of the endocrine system (ductless glands) and houses the optic nerve.

7th Chakra

Related organ:

The cerebrum (upper brain) is the center of reflex movement, emotions and memory.

Related gland:

The pineal produces melatonin, which regulates sleep, mood, puberty and ovarian cycles.

Healing the Body/Mind— Yoga Therapy

Through years of studying raja and hatha yoga, I have developed a personal approach to emotional healing through blending work with the chakras and the asanas. Since 1982, I have used my own brand of yoga therapy in working both privately and in hospitals and treatment centers with adolescents and adults to facilitate the healing of emotional wounds and the rebuilding of broken lives. This chapter, including the list of "Poses To Stimulate Chakras for Emotional Healing," is based on my therapy practice.

Personal practice of yoga should not be considered a substitute for psychotherapy, if there is a genuine need. However, the emotions can be benefited through the careful, conscientious practice of asanas and pranayama, provided one uses them as a vehicle for developing self-knowledge. Self-knowledge is the key to gaining maximum emotional benefit from one's personal practice of yoga. One need always be aware of one's emotional and physical state as part of yoga practice. By refining self-observation one can also learn, for example, how to scan the body to locate weak or imbalanced chakras.

Through intensive study of the nature of the human being, ancient yogis discovered the necessity of keeping a balance between the physical and emotional bodies. They considered the mind to be the driver, which needs to be strong, clear and centered. They viewed the body as a physical vehicle that must be cleansed and purified by removing the energy blocks causing disease. The soul was believed to be the true and eternal identity of human beings, the seat of love and spirituality. According to the system of the yogis, balancing the strength and flexibility of the

body and mind by practicing hatha yoga and pranayama will allow the soul to emerge free from restrictions, keeping it powerful yet centered.

The chakras are housed within the emotional body, and emotional imbalances therefore affect the chakras. At the same time, physical imbalances—whether of glands or internal organs or structures, or from toxins or infectious agents—also affect the chakras. Because of the interconnection of the physical and emotional bodies, we can use asana work to target an area of the body that is weakened to remedy the emotional imbalance. And building a strong emotional body by balancing the chakras will automatically rejuvenate the glands and organs.

A good way to determine whether the chakras are generally functioning properly is to look inward and ask yourself how you feel emotionally and physically. To check on specific chakras, close the eyes and scan the body with the mind's eye. Move through the chakras from the 1st to the 7th.

If it is difficult to get in touch with the energy produced in the area of a chakra, or if it is difficult to envision the color or activity from the chakra, it is imbalanced. If, for example, the mind tries to visualize the seven chakras running up the spine and it is impossible to feel the 2nd or 5th pulsating, it is in need of attention. Find a yoga pose to stimulate that chakra and scan the chakras later to see if the energy flow has increased.

Stimulating the chakras enhances the circulatory and immune systems for proper functioning. The circulatory system consists of the blood, heart, veins and arteries. The immune system includes the lymphatic system, which helps the body fight infections or cancers. This system consists of a network of vessels that drain tissue fluid (lymph) into lymph nodes, larger fluid-containing lymph ducts and specialized organs involved in the immune system. The lymph nodes and organs act as a type of "filter," removing invading organisms or abnormal cells from the lymph fluid and "processing" them in a way that allows the body to fight these harmful agents.

Clustered at strategic points, including the groin, armpits and neck, lymph nodes act similar to drain screens that catch the debris and eliminate bacteria. When infection is apparent, the nodes become inflamed and cause swelling.

The ductless glands pass secretions directly into the blood or lymph and are situated near the centerline of the body. If a gland were not functioning properly, the related chakra would also be affected negatively and vice versa.

The Role of Chakras in Emotional Problems

Energy, grounding, stability. When the mind and body have a difficult time coming together to generate the excitement or energy to get moving, or if it seems impossible to get grounded and balancing is a chore, the 1st chakra needs help to activate the adrenal glands. Standing or seated poses are very helpful for these problems.

Hormones. If sexual drive is imbalanced, creativity or pleasure in life is lacking, or problems are experienced with menstrual periods, the 2nd chakra needs to be focused on. Standing or seated poses are very helpful for this area.

Severe emotional upset. When there is severe emotional upset with a physical feeling like being punched in the stomach, emotions are having a negative impact on many organs: the digestive organs and pancreas. The 3rd chakra at the solar plexus houses the emotional seat and needs attention for healing. Twists or forward bends unblock this area and stimulate the digestive system.

Tightness, heaviness or chronic fatigue. If there is tightness in the throat or difficulty communicating feelings in a positive way, the heart and chest may also feel heavy or closed in. If the metabolism is sluggish, with exhaustion or chronic fatigue, or if the body is holding too much weight, the thyroid may need special attention. Practicing a yoga pose to stimulate the thyroid, thymus and heart, which house the 4th and 5th chakras, would be suggested. Back-bending and inverted poses or twists with the head turned reach these affected areas.

Negativity and chronic emotional imbalance. Feelings of hopelessness, unworthiness, pessimism and the view of life as a glass that is half empty instead of half full indicate that the pituitary and pineal glands as well as the 3rd and 4th chakras are sluggish and need stimulation. Working on increasing positive insight through self-observation and meditation is also in order. Inverted postures and meditating on the 6th and 7th chakras help remedy this negative outlook.

Anxiety, depression, scattered or dull mind. If these symptoms are present, the 6th and 7th chakras, which affect the pituitary and pineal glands, may need a jump-start to get the wheels turning properly for proper mental functioning. Forward bends, balance poses and inverted poses open blocks in the head.

Dissociation. For people who tend to separate mind from body, or who are out of touch with their bodies because of a history of emotional pain, standing or grounding poses are helpful.

"When the senses are stilled, when the mind is at rest,
when the intellect wavers not- then, say the wise,
is reached the highest stage. This steady control of the
senses and mind has been defined as Yoga.
He who attains it is free from delusion."
(The Kathopanishad)

Poses To Stimulate Chakras for Emotional Healing

^^ more difficult poses   * poses renamed or created by author

^^ more difficult poses   * poses renamed or created by author

^^ more difficult poses   * poses renamed or created by author

Yoga Poses for Specific Imbalances

Through shifting cycles of dormancy, growth and change, nature is constantly cleansing and rebalancing itself, destroying and renewing. As the Earth revolves around the Sun, seasons change and nature dictates a long rest for trees, flowers, ground cover and animals. During this resting period, growth subsides and moisture from snow or rains nurtures the Earth for the coming spring and summer. This change of seasons is vital for keeping the Earth balanced and cleansed. Even natural disasters are a cleansing for the Earth, which is constantly shifting and changing.

As human beings living on the planet, we are engaged in the same process on all levels—much more than many realize. Our cellular structure and function shift throughout each day and night. Our bodies are constantly trying to adjust to the daily physical and emotional pressures and long-term stresses of our lives. These stresses cause blocks that prevent energy from flowing or being distributed evenly through proper channels throughout the body. Imbalances and disease—both emotional and physical—are the result. The first step in healing is to educate the mind to recognize discomforts that indicate imbalance in either body or mind. The following poses have proven beneficial with many common problems.

Sluggish Mind
(depression, headache, allergies, colds)

Dolphin Pose, 78–9
Fish Pose, 86–7
^^ Garland Pose, 38–9
^^ Headstand Pose, 34–5
Leo (Lion), Lion Pose, 56–7
^^ Rolling Boat Pose, 7
^^ *Scorpio (Scorpion), Scorpion Prep Pose, 62–3
Shoulderstand Variations, 2–3
^^ Tripod Pose, 32–3
Virgo (Virgin), Child's Pose, 58–9

Stomach Discomfort
(digestive problems, emotional upset)

^^ Balance-on-Wall—Forward Bend Pose, 16
^^ Balance-on-Wall—Twist Pose, 17
*Blossoming Flower (group pose), 25
^^ *Capricorn (Goat), Hands-and-Knees Lift Pose, 66–7
^^ Cow Twist Pose, 18–9
Fish Pose, 86–7
Full Lotus Pose, 23
^^ Garland Pose, 38–9
Half Camel Variation Pose, 15
Half Lotus Pose, 22
*Partner Octopus Pose, 90–1
^^ *Resting Whale Pose, 81
Sagittarius (Archer), Dancer's Pose, 64–5

^^ *Seahorse Pose, 88–9
*Seated Vine Pose, 37
Seated V-Twist Pose, 13
*Snail Pose, 85
Standing Backbend Pose, 14
*Standing Vine Pose, 36
Supine Twist Pose, 12
Waves I: Rolling Situps Pose, 92–3
Waves II: Hands-and-Knees Pose, 94–5
*Whale Pose, 80

Hyperactivity
(all nature poses, especially those working on balance)

*Blossoming Flower (group pose), 25
Forest Trees (group pose), 31
Full Lotus Pose, 23
^^ Garland Pose, 38–9
Half Lotus Pose, 22
^^ Lotus Lift Pose, 24
*Seated Vine Pose, 37
*Standing Vine Pose, 36
^^ *Starfish-on-Wall Pose, 74–5
Tree in Half Lotus Pose, 26–7
^^ Tree in Half Lotus Wrap Pose, 28–9
^^ Tree in Open Leg Twist Pose, 30
^^ Tripod Pose, 32–3

Sleep Disorders

Dolphin Pose, 78–9
Fish Pose, 86–7
Full Lotus Pose, 23
^^ Garland Pose, 38–9
Half Lotus Pose, 22
^^ Headstand Pose, 34–5
Leo (Lion), Lion Pose, 56–7
^^ Pisces (Fish), Fish Leg Lift, 70–1
^^ *Seahorse Pose, 88–9
Seated V-Twist Pose, 13
Shoulderstand Variations, 2–3
*Snail Pose, 85
Supine Twist Pose, 12
^^ Tripod Pose, 32–3

Habitual Emotional Imbalance
(chronic negative outlook on self or life)

Dolphin Pose, 78–9
Fish Pose, 86–7
^^ Garland Pose, 38–9
^^ Headstand Pose, 34–5
Leo (Lion), Lion Pose, 56–7
*Partner Octopus Pose, 90–1
^^ Pisces (Fish), Fish Leg Lift, 70–1
^^ *Resting Whale Pose, 81
^^ Rolling Boat Pose, 7
^^ *Scorpio (Scorpion), Scorpion Prep Pose, 62–3
^^ *Seahorse Pose, 88–9
Seated V-Twist Pose, 13

^^ more difficult poses   * poses renamed or created by author

Dissociation

(tendency to separate mind from body; not being fully in touch with body) standing or grounding poses

PRANAYAMA FOR HEALING

Sluggish Mind

Alternate Nostril Breathing, 42–3
Breath of Fire, 46
Cooling Breath, 44–5
Deep Breathing, 47

Sinus Problems

Alternate Nostril Breathing, 42–3
Cooling Breath, 44–5
Deep Breathing, 47

Anxiety

Abdominal Breathing, 96
Alternate Nostril Breathing, 42–3
Cooling Breath, 44–5
Deep Breathing, 47

Low Energy

Alternate Nostril Breathing, 42–3
Breath of Fire, 46

Sleep Disorders

Alternate Nostril Breathing, 42–3
Cooling Breath, 44–5
Deep Breathing, 47

Depression

Alternate Nostril Breathing, 42–3
Breath of Fire, 46
Cooling Breath, 44–5
Deep Breathing, 47

*"The purpose of Yoga is liberation,
to reach self-understanding
and break bonds of conditioning."*
(Patanjali, Yoga Sutras)

^^ more difficult poses   * poses renamed or created by author

Poses To Strengthen & Stretch Different Areas of the Body

Yoga asanas provide both strengthening and flexibility. In yoga, achieving flexibility goes beyond the focus of the body. Mental flexibility is enhanced by practicing pranayama and by concentrating on the breath to control body movements. The following lists can guide you in selecting poses to strengthen and stretch specific ares of the body.

Upper-Body Strength
(upper back, chest, shoulders, arms, wrists)

*Aries (Ram), Half Warrior III Prep Pose, 48–9
*Cancer (Crab), Crab Pose, 54–5
^^ *Capricorn (Goat), Hands-and-Knees Lift Pose, 66–7
*Crab Walks Race, 84
Dolphin Pose, 78–9
^^ Headstand Pose, 34–5
Leo (Lion), Lion Pose, 56–7
^^ Libra (Balance), Shoulder-and-Arm Balance Pose, 60–1
^^ Lotus Lift Pose, 24
*Partner Octopus Pose, 90–1
Sagittarius (Archer), Dancer's Pose, 64–5
^^* Scorpio (Scorpion), Scorpion Prep Pose, 62–3
*Seal Race with Ball (group pose), 77
Shoulderstand Variations, 2–3
^^ *Starfish-on-Wall Pose, 74–5
Taurus (Bull), Cow's Head Pose, 50–1
^^ Tripod Pose, 32–3

Lower-Body Strength
(hips, legs, ankles)

Aquarius (Water Bearer), Water Wheel Pose, 68–9
*Aries (Ram), Half Warrior III Prep Pose, 48–9
^^ Balance-on-Wall—Forward Bend Pose, 16

^^ Balance-on-Wall—Twist Pose, 17
Boat Pose, 4–5
*Cancer (Crab), Crab Pose, 54–5
^^ *Capricorn (Goat), Hands-and-Knees Lift Pose, 66–7
*Crab Walks Race, 84
Dolphin Pose, 78–9
Fish Pose, 86–7
Forest Trees (group pose), 31
^^ Garland Pose, 38–9
^^ Gemini (Twins), Partner Squats Pose, 52–3
Half Camel Variation Pose, 15
Partner Boat Pose, 6
*Penguin Pose, 82
*Penguin Race (group pose), 83
^^ Pisces (Fish), Fish Leg Lift, 70–1
^^ *Resting Whale Pose, 81
^^ Rolling Boat Pose, 7
^^ Rolling Bow Pose, 10
Sagittarius (Archer), Dancer's Pose, 64–5
^^ *Scorpio (Scorpion), Scorpion Prep Pose, 62–3
^^ *Seahorse Pose, 88–9
*Seal Pose, 76
*Seal Race with Ball (group pose), 77
*Seated Vine Pose, 37
Seated V-Twist Pose, 13
Standing Backbend Pose, 14
*Standing Vine Pose, 36
^^ *Starfish-on-Wall Pose, 74–5
Supine Twist Pose, 12
Tree in Half Lotus Pose, 26–7

^^ Tree in Half Lotus Wrap Pose, 28–9
^^ Tree in Open Leg Twist Pose, 30
Waves I: Rolling Situps Pose, 92–3
Waves II: Hands-and-Knees Pose, 94–5
*Whale Pose, 80

Back-Strengthening Poses

Aquarius (Water Bearer), Water Wheel Pose, 68–9
*Aries (Ram), Half Warrior III Prep Pose, 48–9
^^ Balance-on-Wall—Twist Pose, 17
*Blossoming Flower (group pose), 25
Boat Pose, 4–5
*Cancer (Crab), Crab Pose, 54–5
^^ *Capricorn (Goat), Hands-and-Knees Lift Pose, 66–7
^^ Cow Twist Pose, 18–19
*Crab Walks Race, 84
Dolphin Pose, 78–9
Fish Pose, 86–7
Forest Trees (group pose), 31
Full Lotus Pose, 23
^^ Gemini (Twins), Partner Squats Pose, 52–3
Half Lotus Pose, 22
^^ Headstand Pose, 34–5
Leo (Lion), Lion Pose, 56–7
^^ Libra (Balance), Shoulder-and-Arm Balance Pose, 60–1
^^ Lotus Lift Pose, 24
*Penguin Pose, 82

^^ more difficult poses   * poses renamed or created by author

^^ more difficult poses   * poses renamed or created by author

Sample Workouts

Sample Half-hour Workout

Half Lotus Pose, 22
Alternate Nostril Breathing, 42–3
*Seal Pose, 76
Seated V-Twist Pose, 13
Waves I: Rolling Situps Pose, 92–3
Waves II: Hands-and-Knees Pose, 94–5
*Aries (Ram), Half Warrior III Prep Pose, 48–9
Half Camel Variation Pose, 15
Virgo (Virgin), Child's Pose, 58–9
Tree in Half Lotus Pose. 26–7
Standing Backbend Pose, 14
Sagittarius (Archer), Dancer's Pose, 64–5
^^ Garland Pose, 38–9
Fish Pose, 86–7
*Snail Pose, 85
Relaxation (Savasana), 96

Gentle Half-hour Workout

Begin by standing in Mountain Pose (with Ujjayi Breath [p. 47], 10 deep breaths). Follow with:

Uddiyana Bandha, 11
*Penguin Pose, 82
*Standing Vine Pose, 36
Standing Backbend Pose, 14
Dolphin Pose, 78–9
Taurus (Bull), Cow's Head Pose, 50–1
Leo (Lion) Lion Pose, 56–7
*Whale Pose, 80
*Seal Pose, 76

*Cancer (Crab), Crab Pose, 54–5
Aquarius (Water Bearer), Water Wheel Pose, 68–9
*Snail Pose, 85
Relaxation (Savasana), 96

Intermediate 1-hour Workout

Begin by standing in Mountain Pose (with Ujjayi Breath [p. 47], 5 minutes). Follow with:

*Penguin Pose, 82
*Standing Vine Pose, 36
Standing Backbend Pose, 14
^^ Gemini (Twins), Partner Squats Pose (alone or with partner), 52–3
^^ Garland Pose, 38–9
*Seal Pose, 76
Taurus (Bull), Cow's Head Pose, 50–1
^^ Cow Twist Pose, 18–9
*Seated Vine Pose, 37
Sagittarius (Archer), Dancer's Pose, 64–5
^^ Balance-on-Wall—Forward Bend Pose, 16
^^ Balance-on-Wall—Twist Pose, 17
Aquarius (Water Bearer), Water Wheel Pose, 68–9
Dolphin Pose, 78–9
Virgo (Virgin), Child's Pose, 58–9
*Whale Pose, 80
^^ *Resting Whale Pose, 81
^^ Rolling Bow Pose, 10
*Aries (Ram), Half Warrior III Prep Pose, 48–9
Seated V-Twist Pose, 13

^^ Revolved Head-to-Knee Pose, 8–9
*Cancer (Crab) Crab Pose, 54–5
^^ Headstand Pose, 34–5
Virgo (Virgin), Child's Pose, 58–9
Shoulderstand Variations, 2–3
*Partner Octopus Pose (alone or with partner), 90–1
*Blossoming Flower—Group Pose (alone or with a group), 25
^^ *Seahorse Pose, 88–9
*Snail Pose, 85
Cooling Breath, 44–5
Relaxation (Savasana), 5–10 minutes, 96

Intermediate 1-hour Workout

Half Lotus Pose, 22
Ujjayi Breath, 2–5 minutes, 47
*Seated Vine Pose, 37
*Seal Pose, 76
Full Lotus Pose, 23
^^ Lotus Lift Pose, 24
^^ Garland Pose, 38–9
Tree in Half Lotus Pose, 26–7
^^ Tree in Half Lotus Wrap Pose, 28–9
Sagittarius (Archer), Dancer's Pose, 64–5
Waves I: Rolling Situps Pose, 92–3
^^ *Capricorn (Goat), Hands-and-Knees Lift Pose, 66–7
^^ Libra (Balance), Shoulder-and-Arm Balance Pose, 60–1
^^ Revolved Head-to-Knee Pose, 8–9

^^ more difficult poses   * poses renamed or created by author

116

^^ more difficult poses   * poses renamed or created by author

Group Poses for Children & Teens

Children will be intrigued by the poses in this book relating to Nature. For ages of 3–12, it is important to focus on strengthening all parts of the body, especially the abdominal and back muscles. A notation with each pose gives the appropriate age for the beginning of its practice. As with any physical exercises, it is important for children to learn the poses from qualified teachers, preferably adults.

The group poses or races are great fun and highly beneficial in building motor skills and concentration. It is important for children to learn to practice each pose alone first to understand its dynamics relating to proper alignment before they work on movement with the pose.

Young children ages 3–10 will not need to practice Pranayama, bandhas or chakra work yet, since the chakras are still developing.

Teenagers will benefit from the poses to build both strength and flexibility of the body and mind, enhancing concentration skills for school work or interactive sports. The partner poses, group poses or races help solidify social skills by interaction with others.

Group Poses to Practice:

Forest Trees (group pose), 31
*Blossoming Flower (group pose), 25
*Seal Race with Ball (group pose), 77
*Crab Walks Race, 84
*Penguin Race (group pose), 83
*Partner Octopus Pose, 90–1
Partner Boat Pose, 6
^^ Gemini (Twins), Partner Squats Pose, 52–3

^^ more difficult poses   * poses renamed or created by author

Epilogue

Sanskrit Glossary

Pronunciation Guide

a as in up	*ṅ* as in encore	*ś* as in tissue
ā as in father	*ṇ* as in friend	*ṣ* as in hush
ch as in coach	*o* as in boy	*ṭ* as in cart
i as in city	*ṛ* as in sabre	*ū* as in rule
ī as in petite	*ṝ* as in chagrin	*u* as in bull
e as in meeting		

Anguṣṭa—big toe

Apāna—vital air of lower abdomen

Ardha—half

Āsana—posture

Baddha—bound, caught, restrained

Bandha—bondage, a posture where organs or parts of the body are contracted or controlled.

Bhuja—the shoulder or arm

Bhujang—cobra

Dhānu—a bow

Dharana—one of the eight limbs of raja yoga, concentration

Dhyana—one of the eight limbs of raja yoga, meditation

Gomukha—face resembling a cow

Guṇa—a quality or ingredient of nature

Hala—a plow

Hasta—the hand

Hatha—(*ha*–sun and *tha*–moon), the first path of yoga (physical discipline)

Jālandhara—a posture where the neck and throat are contracted and the chin rests in the notch between the collarbones at the top of the breast bone (chin lock), one of the three bandhas

Jānu—the knee

Jaṭhara—the abdomen, stomach

Jnāna—true knowledge

Kapālabhāti (*kāpola*–skull, *bhāti*–light, luster)—a process of clearing and strengthening the lungs and mind

Kona—angle

Kūrma—a tortoise

Lola—swing

Mālā—a garland, wreath

Matsya—a fish

Mayūra—a peacock

Mudrā—a sealing posture, external closing of fingers, arms

Mūla—the root, base

Nāṭarāja—a name of Siva, the lord of the dancers

Nāva—a boat

Pāda—foot or leg

Pādma—a lotus

Parivartana—turning around, revolved

Parivṛtta—turned around, revolved

Pārṣva—the side, flank, lateral

Pīdā—pressure

Pinda—fetus or embryo, body

Prāna—breath, respiration, life, vitality, wind, energy, strength. It also means the "soul."

Pranayama—breath control

Prasārita—stretched out

Pratayahara—one of the eight limbs of raja yoga, drawing the senses inward

Pūrva—the east side, front side of the body

Pūrvottana—the intense stretch of the front side of the body

Sālamba—with support

Samadhi—one of the eight limbs of raja yoga, a state in which the aspirant is one with the object of his meditation, as a Supreme Spirit connecting with the Universe, a feeling of extreme joy and peace

Śava—a corpse, dead body

Sarvāṅa—the whole body

Sattva—the pure and good quality of everything in nature, one of the three qualities of energy in nature

Siṃha—a lion

Sirṣa—the head

Supta—sleeping, lying down

Sutra—thread

Tāda—mountain

Tamas—darkness or ignorance, one of the three qualities of energy in nature

Tola—a balance

Uḍḍīyāna—bondage, the diaphragm is lifted high up the thorax and the abdominal organs are pulled back toward the spine. When holding *Uḍḍīyāna Bandha*, the great bird Prana (life) is forced to fly up through the Sushumna nadi.

Ujjayi—a type of pranayama where the lungs are fully expanded and the chest is puffed out

Upaviṣṭha—seated

Ūrdhva—raised, elevated, tending upward

Utkaṭa—powerful, fierce

Uttāna—an intense stretch

Utthiṭa—raised, extended, stretched

Vīrabhadra—a powerful hero created out of Siva's matted hair

Vasiṣṭha—a celebrated sage, author of several Vedic hymns

Vṛkṣa—a tree

Vṛśchika—a scorpion

Yama—control

Bibliography

Sacred Classical Texts Used by the Author

Bhagavad Gita. The most important authority on yoga philosophy, this includes the story of Lord Krishna's instruction of warrior Arjuna in yoga, teachings on how to achieve liberation by fulfilling one's duties in life.

Vedas. A vast collection of scriptures dating as far back as 2500 B.C.

Upanishads. Forming the later sections of the Vedas, these provide the main foundation of yoga teaching. They incorporate the philosophy known as Vedanta, which is based on the concept of one absolute reality or consciousness, known as Brahman, which underlies all existence.

Yoga Sutras, by Patanjali. Written in the 3rd century B.C., this is a description of the science of yoga and the backbone of raja yoga. It consists of 195 sutras divided into sections addressing the nature of the body and its treatment, the nature of thoughts and their place in the process of living, the nature of consciousness, and the nature of the breath and its control.

Hatha Yoga Pradipika, by Swatmarama. This describes the various asanas and breathing exercises that form the basis of the modern practice of yoga.

Other Source Books Used by the Author

Atlas of the Human Body. New York: Harper Perennial Book, 1994.

Herring, Barbara Kaplan. "Seventh Heaven." Yoga Journal. December 2001.

Iyengar, B.K.S. Light on Yoga. New York: Shocken Books, 1979.

Kraftsow, Gary. Yoga for Wellness. New York: The Penguin Group, 1999.

Little, Marjorie. The Endocrine System. Philadelphia: Chelsea House Publishers, 2001.

McAfee, John. Secrets of the Yamas. Woodland Park, Col.: Woodland Publications, 2001.

Sivananda Yoga Center. The Sivananda Companion to Yoga. New York: Simon & Schuster, 2000.

Stiles, Mumunda, interp. Yoga Sutras by Patanjali. Boston: Red Wheel/Weiser, LLC., 2002.

ABOUT THE AUTHOR

Thia Luby was introduced to yoga in 1971 by her older brother, when he returned home during a college break. This brief experience sparked an interest in yoga and a lifelong journey. In 1972 Luby began intensive practice of different paths of yoga as well as in-depth research in the field. This personal path became a full-time career in 1978 and has continued to blossom through three decades.

Luby has devoted her time to a wide spectrum of students. Her teaching began with adults and progressed into prenatal, children and teens, all in diverse settings. Since the 1980s she has focused on teaching yoga in the psychological field, working in hospitals and treatment centers.

Her daughter, Bianca, was raised on yoga and helped teach children's classes for years. Luby now has two young grandchildren to whom she is introducing the fun and benefits of yoga practice.

Luby is the author of two other yoga books. *Children's Book of Yoga* won a national award from *School Library Journal* as one of the best children's books of 1998. Her second book, *Yoga for Teens,* received an honorable mention from *School Library Journal* and an enthusiastic response from *Teen Magazine.*

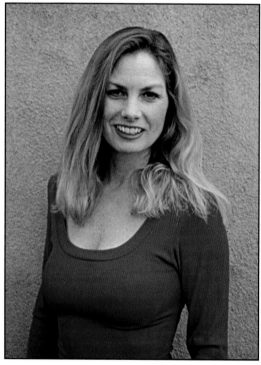

photo ©Marcia Keegan

122

A Note from the Author

My twenty-plus years of working with adolescents and adults in emotional healing and life rebuilding has touched me deeply, especially when being thanked by so many clients who honor my work as new and different from anything they have experienced before. For both those in my private practice and those in hospitals and treatment centers, these yoga therapy sessions become key components in their recovery programs.

The following experience illustrates how my yoga therapy works. One of my clients, about to be discharged, felt happy to be leaving the facility soon and building a new life, yet at the same time he felt remorse, sadness and fear around leaving new friends and an important support system, which was monumental in his recovery. He had a stomach ache and tightness in the chest.

After deliberating, it was apparent he needed work on balancing the 1st chakra for grounding energy to help him "out the door" without looking back with any regrets or negative emotions. His 3rd and 4th chakras were the other two important chakras that needed balancing. His "emotional seat" was teetering and stirring upset in his stomach from fear and remorse. His "heart center" was torn from sadness and hurt over leaving a lot behind.

We worked on Tree Poses to help him bring the energy down into the 1st chakra and become more rooted. At the same time, we worked on opening the 3rd and 4th chakras with more poses featuring the opening of the chest. While holding each pose, I asked him to focus on opening the heart center and emotional seat and feel rooted so he could take all the positives "on the road" with him to get rooted elsewhere, away from this facility. I also asked him to keep his peers in his heart with warm thoughts and to release the fear in his belly by turning it into a powerful light to guide his new journey. We also worked on Boat Pose, Seated V-Twist Pose, Supine Twist Pose and Shoulderstand Variations.

Focusing on all three chakras at once helped to bring him into a balanced state of awareness and aided him in "letting go" of the negative energy blocked in those areas.

He felt all the pain and fear subside. I had worked with him regularly for one month, and he was amazed at the positive effects of this new yoga therapy he had experienced with me. It was heart-warming for me to be able to send him on his way with new information he can use for his entire lifetime. He was hooked on yoga!